LIFELONG YOUTH

THE SIMPLE PATH TO A LONG & YOUTHFUL LIFE

Parker Hewes, DC

D1534054

i

Deb,

So happy to be part of your health journey! Keep up the good work

Stay Young!

Follow Us!

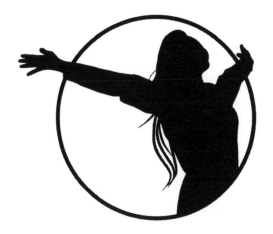

Web: lifelongyouthbook.com

facebook.com/LifelongYouth

instagram.com/mylifelongyouth/

First paperback edition May 2021

Book design by Parker Hewes
Cover design by Parker Hewes

ISBNs: 9798702966267

For more information:
Website: lifelongyouthbook.com
Email: mylifelongyouth@gmail.com

A message for the reader:
The contents of this book are for informational purposes only. It does not constitute medical advice, and is not intended to be a substitute for, or replace professional medical advice, diagnosis, or treatment. Always seek the advice of a physician or other qualified health provider with any questions you may have regarding a medical condition, and before following or relying upon any information in this book. Never disregard professional medical advice or delay in seeking it because of something you have read in this book. The authors and publishers specifically disclaim all responsibility for any liability, loss, or risk, personal or otherwise, which is incurred as a consequence, directly or indirectly, of the use and application of any of the contents of this book. The reader of this material is responsible for his or her own actions and conclusions.

This book is dedicated to my childhood, including my mom, dad, sister, friends, parents of friends, relatives, teachers, coaches, and classmates. You all afforded me so much happiness and joy. Because of you, I was inspired to write this book about maintaining the youthfulness in all of us.

Also, to my future children, I am so excited to be your father, playing games, and enjoying life with you until I'm laid to rest.

Table of Contents

Part III: The Simple Steps

FOREWORD:

A NOTE ON RESEARCH

This book is based on scientific research, but research is not perfect.

First, human behaviors are highly variable, so it is difficult to do research that controls all those variables. And even if we could control every variable, the way your body responds could be drastically different from how the research participants responded. At various stages of life, your body has different physiologic responses, too.

Second, diet and lifestyle research relies mostly on epidemiological data. This means that the study results can only show associations; it cannot tell us that one thing directly caused something else. For example, there is an association between exercise and longevity, but that does not mean that exercise *causes* longevity.

Third, we perform a lot of nutritional research on animals. Animal studies give us a lot of knowledge about basic science and biochemistry, but we cannot be sure that the effect will be the same in humans. We shouldn't discredit animal research entirely, but we ought to be critical.

Additionally, some of the knowledge in this book comes from non-scientific sources. For example, observing the behaviors of healthy or long-living cultures can give us some insight into how to live. After all, healthy cultures have been proving their methods for hundreds of years. They may not have published their work, but I'm not going to discredit Joe Caveman just because he isn't cited in JAMA (Journal of the American Medical Association). Humans have been tinkering with not dying for our entire existence, which means we have thousands of years of trial and error under our belts. If you ask me, that makes for a pretty convincing case, maybe even better than a scientific paper.

To summarize, you should know that the ideas in this book are not my own. Rather, this book is an aggregation of knowledge from the brilliant people that came before me. If anything in this book appears useful or clever, you can attribute it to those people. If anything seems foolish or somewhat silly, you can attribute it to me.

Introduction

Ugh, not another book about health. What more could I possibly say?

Honestly, not much. You already know how to be healthy; there is just so much noise in the health world that it's hard to know which behaviors are the most important. You try to listen to the advice of health gurus, experts, journalists, scientists, and doctors, but they all seem to be saying something different. Your doctor tells you to wash your hands religiously, but you heard something about your microbiome on the news last week - they said that bacteria is *healthy* for you.

So, which is it? Should you be washing the dirt off your hands or smearing it on your face? You might as well eat it while you're at it, right?

It's okay. You are not alone in your confusion. Thankfully, there is a way out. Grab your machete and your rubber boots because we are going to sift through this jungle together. When you hack away the mess of overgrown brambles and bushes, you'll see that there is a clear path to health. I'm here to help you find it.

ALERT:
Some people don't want to learn about all the scientific
details; they just want "how-to" descriptions. If you feel the
same way, turn to Part III.
I get it, no hard feelings.

CHAPTER 1:

LIFESPAN VS. HEALTHSPAN

Five signs that you're turning 50

1. Your back goes out more than you do.
2. You're in the elevator, and your favorite song comes on.
3. People start telling you how good you look for your age.
4. You can fart, sneeze, and pee at the same time.
5. The candles cost more than the birthday cake.

Today, 50 is considered "over the hill," but in 1900, America's average life expectancy was 49. Since then, modern medicine has mastered the science of treating infectious diseases, performing emergency care, and diminishing infant mortality, which has raised our life expectancy to 78.6.[1] From 2000 to 2016, we saw the fastest increase in life expectancy since the 1960s.[2]

Then, the trend reversed. After 2016, life expectancy declined, and it declined every year for the following three years. Now, for the first time in history, we expect today's generation of kids to live shorter lifespans than their parents.[3]

I'll admit, this drop in life expectancy could be a fluke or a result of the opioid crisis. Still, I wonder if we have hit the cap. Could it be that we have reached the limit on how long our medical system can keep us alive?

David Sinclair would argue that we have the genetic fortitude to live to age 120. But how good will those extra years be if we are bedridden or stuck in a nursing home? Maybe it's time to focus on another aspect of life. Perhaps we should worry about the quality of our life, not just the length of it. Instead of trying to lengthen our lifespan, let's strive to be healthy, vibrant, and youthful for as long as possible. Some call this healthspan; I call it lifelong youth.

CHAPTER 2:

PHYSICAL, MENTAL, & SOCIAL WELL-BEING

"Health is a state of complete physical, mental, and social well-being and not merely the absence of disease or infirmity."
- World Health Organization

Read that quote again. It says that health is NOT just the absence of disease. Health is a state of well-being. The word "well-being" is a little vague, though, because it means something different to each person. So, I describe well-being as a simple equation.

Well-being = more positive experiences than negative ones.

Whether we are talking about physical, mental, or social well-being, the equation stays the same. When you add positive behaviors, positive thoughts, and positive interactions to your life, you tilt the scales in favor of well-being.

In the case of mental and social health, your chance to improve your well-being is unlimited. The number of positive or negative thoughts that you have in a lifetime is endless, and if you make a conscious effort to be more positive than negative, you are more likely to achieve well-being. Likewise, your social interactions can be as positive as you want them to be. Every interaction is an opportunity to have a positive experience, and there is no limit to how close, connected, and happy you could feel around others.

Thankfully, you don't need to be a beaming light of positivity all the time; that would be dishonest. But if you strive to be generally more positive than negative, you will have a ripple effect bigger than you can imagine.

Physical well-being, on the other hand, is not unlimited. Your muscles can't grow forever, your stomach can't fit infinite food, and you probably can only live to be 120 tops (122 is the record).

However, you can think, learn, and choose behaviors that will optimize your physical well-being. It may seem like a lot of work, but the path to health is paved with steppingstones. You don't need to scale the mountain in a single bound; you just need to put one foot in front of the other. So, let's walk this trail together.

Part I
What Determines Your Health?

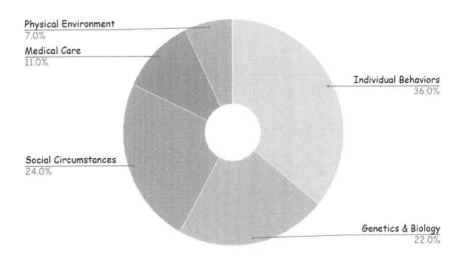

Physical Environment
7.0%

Medical Care
11.0%

Individual Behaviors
36.0%

Social Circumstances
24.0%

Genetics & Biology
22.0%

CHAPTER 3:

YOU DO

"There is no I in Team, but there is a You in Youth."
- Parker Hewes

It should come as no surprise that your health is in your hands. We are talking about **your** health, after all, so **YOU** are the most important factor.

In Steven Covey's bestselling book, <u>The Seven Habits of Highly Effective People</u>, he illustrates the power of YOU by explaining the difference between your circle of concern, circle of influence, and circle of control.

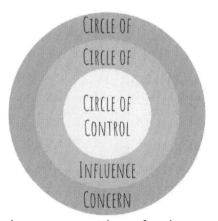

Your circle of concern includes all the worries you have in life (kids, work, taxes, the threat of war, politics, etc.), while your circle of control only pertains to the concerns directly within your control. Your circle of control is much smaller than your circle of concern (see image to the right), primarily because many things are out of your control. For example, you may be concerned that it will rain tomorrow, but you can't do anything about it, so it is out of your control. You can, however, control your preparedness for the inclement weather by putting on a rain jacket. Putting on a rain jacket, then, would fall in your circle of control.

It is no use worrying about the things in your circle of concern if you can't actually do anything about them. Worrying will just add unnecessary stress to your life. A highly effective person still has concerns, but their worries get them to take action and control what they can. Any extra worrying is deemed unnecessary and likely harmful to their productivity, happiness, and health. Thus, you have a choice. You can dwell on all the concerns you have in life, or you can focus on only those within your control. If you dwell on the problems that are not in your control, you will likely become distracted, frustrated, and stressed. Also, as you will see in the following pages, dwelling on the concerns that are out of your control will cause your circle of influence to shrink, thus making you a less effective person overall and less likely to achieve your goals.

To further explain this point, let's look at the differences between a reactive and proactive person.

The **reactive person** worries about things that they can't control. They are always reacting to outside forces, so their time is occupied by worrying instead of doing.

Reactive people use "ifs and have's" in their language. They say things like, "If I had ___, then I would be healthier. If the government would do ___, then ___. If my boss were more ___, then I would like my job. I'll be happy when someone does ___."

Since reactive people focus on worrying instead of doing, their behaviors are inefficient, and their circle of influence shrinks (see image on the right). They can barely keep their personal affairs in order, let alone influence someone else.

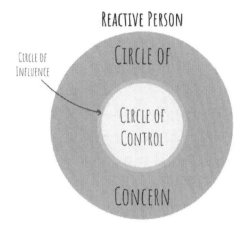

The **proactive person**, on the other hand, takes responsibility for their own life. They work on things that are within their control and thus increase their circle of influence.

Proactive people use "be" in their language. They say things like, "I can be better at ___. I can be more ___. I can do ___."

Since proactive people focus on things within their control, they are more efficient with their time and energy. Instead of spending their time waiting for someone else to make a move, proactive people do what they can to affect the desired outcome.

Regarding your health, being a proactive person means focusing on the behaviors that you can control. As you will see in the next chapter, many factors influence your health, but that does not mean you have to worry about all of them. However, for almost every factor that impacts your health, you can do something to be proactive and effective. And most of the time, these healthy choices will echo throughout your community, illustrating how you can expand your circle of influence by focusing on your circle of control.

CHAPTER 4:

DETERMINANTS OF HEALTH[4]

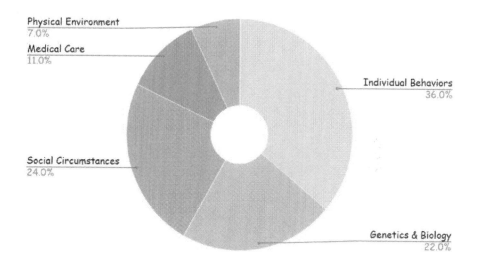

Physical Environment
7.0%

Medical Care
11.0%

Individual Behaviors
36.0%

Social Circumstances
24.0%

Genetics & Biology
22.0%

According to the world's leading public health organizations[5], five overarching factors determine your health. These determinants include:

1. Physical environment (7%)
2. Medical care (11%)
3. Social circumstances (24%)
4. Genetics & biology (22%)
5. Individual behaviors (36%)

According to the researchers, some determinants occupy a bigger percentage of the health pie, so they impact your health more than others. But no matter how you slice it, only one category is 100% within your circle of control, your individual behaviors.

The other determinants may be in your circle of concern, but you can't totally control them. You can't force mother nature to grow more trees (physical environment) or tell your parents what genes to give to you (genetics & biology). You also can't control how much education your doctor received (medical care) or if your town is vibrant and social (social circumstances).

However, you can still influence these determinants of health by focusing on your individual behaviors (aka your circle of control). In doing so, you will connect the pieces of the pie like a Venn-Diagram, with your individual behaviors acting as the glue that holds it all in place.

DETERMINANTS OF HEALTH

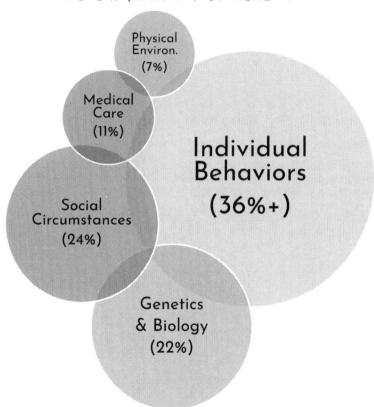

In the following pages, I give some examples of how your individual behaviors can influence the other four determinants of health. For each determinant, I zoom in on the smaller subcategories, which are called micro-determinants.

As you look through the flow charts, see if you can start connecting the dots between your individual behaviors and the micro-determinants. Try to come up with a couple of examples of how your behaviors might be influential.

Also, feel free to come up with your own micro-determinants of health. After all, the flow charts do not represent an exhaustive list. Health is a very complex topic, and these oversimplified flow charts are only meant to provide a framework.

MICRO-DETERMINANTS OF HEALTH REGARDING YOUR PHYSICAL ENVIRONMENT.

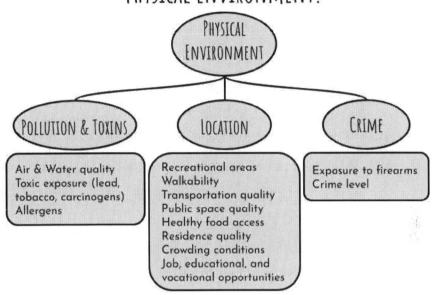

The physical environment around you (such as toxins, crime, housing quality, and public parks) can affect your ability to perform healthy behaviors. For example, if your town doesn't have sidewalks and there are a lot of allergens in the air, you probably won't be going for walks very often. Similarly, if there is more crime in your area, your fear will cause unhealthy stress, and you will likely spend more time indoors.

Topics like sidewalk construction or crime reduction may be in your circle of concern, but they are not in your circle of control. Moving to a new location is within your control, but that is difficult for most people. Instead, you might consider improving your physical environment by cleaning up parks, taking care of your residence, or serving on a local public health council.

You could also try minimizing your environmental impact by composting, conserving water, recycling, or using renewable fuel. After all, ecological health translates into individual health. Try going for a run in Los Angeles when the smog rolls in, and you'll see what I mean.

Even if you don't care about environmental causes, healthy behaviors will still benefit ecosystem health. For example, eating local, organic foods is correlated with better health. At the same time, local and organic foods have a smaller ecological footprint because the food doesn't travel as many miles to get to your dinner table.

Below are some more ways to improve your health and reduce your ecological footprint at the same time:

- Use renewable energy (solar, wind, and other high-efficiency energy sources). Renewable energy produces nearly zero pollution.
- Eat locally. Our current model of industrial agriculture is energetically expensive. Buying from local farmers reduces the amount of fuel required to transport and store your food. Plus, local food is probably raised more humanely and is less likely to have unwanted preservatives, pesticides, hormones, and antibiotics.
- Ditch the car; walk and bike more. Use muscle power to drastically improve your full-body health while also reducing your dependence on fuels.
- Vote with your wallet. By supporting businesses that share your values of reducing waste and pollution, you create a precedent so other companies will follow suit. It also sets an example for you to reduce your household waste.

Side Note: The Role of Public Health

As you look through this first flow chart, you may be thinking, "I can't do anything about that; these categories are too big for one person to change." I think you are right. While there are still plenty of small actions that can have huge effects, some things require collective action. In my opinion, that is where public health comes in. Public health's role is to address the micro-determinants of health within our circle of concern, but not entirely in our control.

The public health department doesn't have to make grand, elaborate changes, though. By paying attention to civic design, culture, and green space, your government can create an environment that gently nudges people to be happier and healthier. Instead of forcing health on people, public health can make small changes in the community, so the healthy option is more accessible, safer, prettier, and enticing. Like a subliminal message, people will choose healthy behaviors without even realizing it. Health becomes the default option.

*One thing **you** can do is get involved in your public health department. Your opinion can make a big difference.*

The Micro-Determinants of Health Regarding Medical Care.

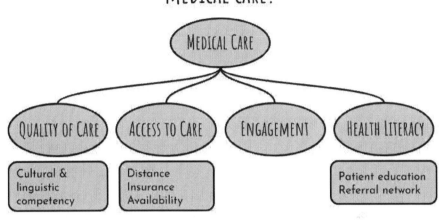

We put a lot of trust in medical care when it comes to our health, but medical care only plays a small role in determining your health.

Most of your life is spent outside of the doctor's office, anyway, so we shouldn't rely on our doctors to keep us healthy. As Hippocrates would say, "the greatest medicine of all is to teach people how not to need it."

Sometimes you're going to need medical care, though. If that day comes, your doctors must be easily accessible, engaged in your community, connected to other providers, and committed to enhancing your health literacy. These characteristics describe a high-quality doctor, and everyone should have access to this kind of medical care.

You have no control over the medical system's caliber, but your individual behaviors can still have an impact. For instance, when you have healthy behaviors, you get sick less, and you won't *need* to see a doctor as often. But healthy people know that preventing a problem is far cheaper and more effective than reacting to one. So, instead of *needing* a doctor to fix your disease, you'll *want* to see a doctor, even when you feel perfectly healthy.

With this type of attitude, you can take your time to look for a high-quality provider. In doing so, you elevate the entire medical profession because you reward good doctors with your business. Meanwhile, the lower caliber doctors are motivated to be better so they can keep their job.

The micro-determinants of health regarding your social circumstances.

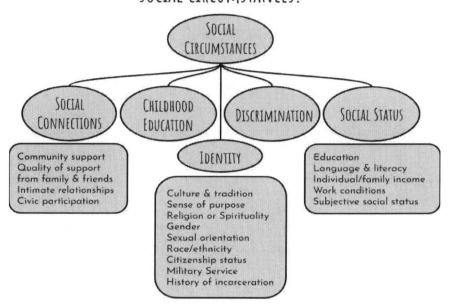

Humans are one of the most social creatures on Earth. It is no wonder that our social circumstances are a significant determinant of health. Our inter-connectedness helped our species become smarter, more efficient, and (dare I say) happier.

But we all know that our social interactions can also be stressful and unhealthy. In these situations, taking control of your individual behaviors will help you weather the storm.

Even if it is someone else's "fault," I implore you to focus on your own behaviors and not worry about the actions of others (which are out of your control).

For example, if you have a frustrating social experience (i.e., discrimination), you can decide to respond positively instead of negatively. Or you can choose to move on and put the bad experience behind you. Be the bigger person, as they say.

You can also improve your social connectedness by joining a civic group, starting a club, or investing in your existing relationships.

Finally, if you want to improve your social status, you can choose to get out there and learn. Knowledge is free, and everyone has the same amount of time in their day. By spending your time studying useful information, you can improve your income, social status, and, ultimately, your health.

THE MICRO-DETERMINANTS OF HEALTH REGARDING YOUR GENETICS AND BIOLOGY.

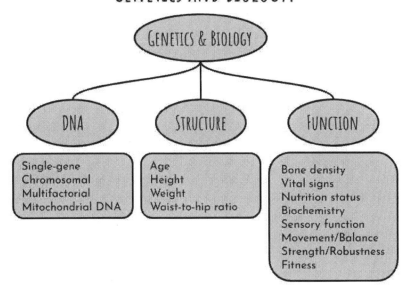

This may seem crazy to you, but you can change your genetics and biology. Okay, maybe not your age and height, but everything else is totally within your control.

For example, your genes are not fixed; they can be turned on, turned off, repaired, or replaced. Therefore, you don't need to worry so much about your genetic predisposition for disease. Even if everyone in your family has heart disease, that does not mean you will inevitably get heart disease; it just means that your heart is probably a weak link. With this valuable knowledge, you can now focus on the individual behaviors that help strengthen your heart.

And thankfully, it often won't matter where you have a weak link. Practicing healthy behaviors will help you combat any disease, not just the one that runs in your family. By choosing the right behaviors, you can change your whole body's structure and function, thus keeping you feeling strong, vibrant, and disease-free, even into your 80's and 90's.

PART II
ACTIVATING YOUR INNER
"YOUNGIN"

If you like to ask questions about how something works or why it works, this part is for you. If you don't care how your body works, go ahead and skip to Part III. However, some of the information in this section will help you understand the charts in Part III. If you're confused, come on back to the ole' Part Deux, and we'll get you up to speed.

In the meantime, the scientific brains of the world will be over here, getting nerdy about the wondrous inner workings of this crazy vessel we call the human body.

Also, for the remainder of this book, I will be referring to four mechanisms of lifelong youth.

1. Your self-regulatory systems, which keep your body functioning normally.
2. Your structure & mobility, which keeps your body moving smoothly and fluidly.
3. Your self-healing systems, which help revitalize your vulnerable tissues.
4. Your stress management capabilities, which allow you to limit harmful stress and maximize helpful stress.

These mechanisms are highly simplified, and they do not explain everything that is going on inside you. But, by preserving the quality of these life-giving systems, you will master the fundamentals of lifelong youth.

CHAPTER 5:

SELF-REGULATING SYSTEMS

The human body is just a pile of cells. 37.2 trillion, to be exact. And every single one of those cells has a specific role in the body. Some cells are skin cells, while others are liver cells, muscle cells, nerve cells, etc.

Cells are like your employees. When one cell is unhealthy, it will not perform its job as well. If many cells are under-performing, an entire branch of your business (a.k.a. your organs) will under-perform. Since every organ employs billions of cells, it takes a lot of bad cells before you start to notice organ dysfunction. Plus, your body is so good at adapting that you can go on living for a long time without ever knowing that something was amiss.

But, if your cells continue to underperform for years, you'll start to feel the effects. Some people may feel "a little off," while others might notice that they can't do things the way they used to. All too often, though, cellular dysfunction shows up as organ failure, disease, or death.

If you want to ensure that your little employees are at peak performance, you must give them the attention they deserve. When you treat your body well, you give your cells a healthy work environment. And with the right environment, your cells can perform their basic functions happily, energetically, and productively.

Lucky for you, you don't need to do different things to take care of your skin cells, liver cells, nerve cells, and so on. The essential functions of all cells are quite similar, so the same basic behaviors will benefit any cell type. The essential cellular functions include:

Assimilation
Energy production
Communication
Transport

Cells also need to heal and protect themselves, but we will cover those topics in the self-healing chapter.

Assimilation & Energy Production

For a cell to do its job, it needs energy and amino acids. Cells use energy to build things. They mainly build proteins, which are essential for every function in your body. The building blocks for proteins are amino acids. With energy and amino acids, your cells could perform any job that they want.

But to make energy and protein, cells need vitamins (K, A, D, E, B-vitamins, and C), minerals (choline, calcium, magnesium, potassium, sodium, iron, zinc, copper, chromium, iodine, selenium, and fluoride), and oxygen. Getting oxygen is easy; all you need to do is breathe. Adequate nutrition, though, is a bit more of a challenge.

Your body can make some nutrients on its own, but many nutrients need to be ingested. So, an improper diet can easily throw off your nutrient balance. Researchers estimate that over 1/3 of the world is malnourished because they are not getting the nutrients necessary to maintain the essential functions of a cell.[6]

However, many people are malnourished because they are not absorbing their nutrients properly. The ability of cells to absorb nutrients is called assimilation. You can have the best diet in the world, but if you are not absorbing the nutrients from your food, you will still be dysfunctional. In the microbiome chapter, you will learn how imbalanced gut flora can lead to malabsorption and cell dysfunction.

Communication & Transport

Your cells also need to communicate with each other. Without communication, your heart would pump irregularly, your muscles would twitch and seize, your mind wouldn't think straight, and your whole body would be uncoordinated. Maybe you know someone with these miscommunication problems; doctors call it atrial fibrillation, muscular dystrophy, or Alzheimer's disease.

These disorders are the result of severe communication problems. However, even small amounts of miscommunication can cause cellular dysfunction. Once enough cells start getting the wrong message, entire organs may start malfunctioning.

Your body's transport systems are crucial for communication, too. The central communication highways in your body are your nerves and blood vessels. Your nerves can carry a message from the tip of your toe, up to your brain, and back again. Meanwhile, your blood vessels carry hormones that create systemic changes in your body.

Nerves and vessels do more than just transport messages, though. They carry nutrients, proteins, and oxygen, all of which are necessary for maintaining cellular function. They also carry immune cells and antibodies to protect and defend your body, but more on that later.

CHAPTER 6:
BODY STRUCTURE & MOBILITY

Movement is life. Every living thing must be able to move to survive. Plants need to move in the wind, or else they would get knocked down and die. Animals need to move to find food and avoid predators. And your body needs to move, so it doesn't break down. Without movement, your body thinks, "Hey, I'm not using these muscles and joints; I must not need them." It will start taking proteins and calcium away from your bones, muscles, and joints and use the energy in other parts of your body. The result is osteoporosis, sarcopenia, and early death.

Preventing sarcopenia (aka muscle loss) is one of the key indicators for longevity, which is one reason why you should consume *more* protein as they get older, not less. Maintaining your muscle mass is also an indicator of happiness as you age. Stronger muscles allow you to move independently, travel, and play. Conversely, weak muscles increase your likelihood of falling, breaking a bone, and ending up in a nursing home because you can no longer independently care for yourself. People who break a hip in their elder years often end up dying in a nursing home after 3-5 years, partly due to their loss of independence and their immobility.[7]

Movement is also a healing activity. For example, your muscles help pump fluid through your veins and lymph vessels. This pumping action pushes immune cells through your body and increases your resilience against infection. Also, by frequently moving, you will be clearing out waste from your tissues and rejuvenating your body and mind like a crisp, clean river. If you are immobile, stagnant ponds of fluid in your body will become breeding grounds for infection and disease.

The key to movement health is variety. If you move in many unique ways, without compensation or struggle, you will maintain your youthfulness. Just like a child, you will be more flexible, agile, and resilient against injury. Also, you will preserve your independence because you can perform any task that your daily life requires.

In general, humans should be able to walk, run, jump, squat, lunge, crawl, bend, twist, carry, climb, push, pull, lift, throw, and hang. But more specifically, scientists and doctors have identified a list of unique movements that act as indicators of structural health and movement integrity.

These movements are called "fundamental patterns" because they are foundational to most of your activities of daily living. Therefore, if you want to retain your independence and freedom, you should maintain these movement competencies for most of your life. To borrow a phrase from Kelly Starrett, these are like "movement vital signs," and they include:

1. Belly breathing
2. Ground get up
3. Toe-touch
4. Deep squat
5. Hurdle step
6. In-line lunge
7. Active straight leg raise
8. Standing/seated rotation
9. Wall angel
10. Trunk stability push-up
11. Rotary stability
12. Y-balance

Whether you are a high-level athlete or pursuing the athletics of being human, maintaining these baseline movements will help you avoid injury and sustain your youthful mobility for longer.

In the "Mobility Check-up" addendum, you'll find a more detailed description of each of these movement vital signs. To keep track of your movement health, you can perform the mobility check-up on a monthly or yearly basis.

CHAPTER 7:

SELF-HEALING SYSTEMS

Imagine living your whole life in a spacesuit. This space suit protects you from every possible sickness or injury. You have never sprained an ankle, had an infection, gotten a bruise, or experienced emotional distress. Nothing. In terms of being disease-free, you are entirely healthy.

But one day, you decide that you want to step outside that space suit and experience the world with your own hands. So, you take off one glove and press your fingers into a lush bed of grass.

Ow! Your skin is so fragile from being in the spacesuit that the grass has cut your finger, and it drew blood. In a few days, your finger swells with infectious pus. A week later, you're dead.

How could this be? You've never been sick in your entire life. How can a silly cut be so damaging?

The problem is the spacesuit. Your body relied on the protection of the spacesuit for your whole life, so it never had to build up any of its own defenses. By shielding yourself from the dangers of the world, you made your body *more* susceptible to the dangers of the world. A small cut and a few bacteria were enough to kill you because your body wasn't prepared for the insult.

Thankfully, you don't live in a spacesuit. You live in the real world, where you get infected, injured, battered, and bruised regularly. In response to these insults, your body has developed ways to keep you alive and well. I call it self-healing, and you need it to live a long and youthful life.

Your body uses six major systems to heal itself.[8]
1. The microbiome
2. Your immune system and inflammation
3. Angiogenesis
4. DNA protection and repair
5. Cell regeneration
6. Detoxification and excretion.

We will discuss each of these systems in greater detail so you can understand why it is vital to maintain their function.

MICROBIOME

In your gut, on your skin, and throughout your body, billions of bacteria are living peacefully inside you. Your body is like an ecosystem, a rainforest with thousands of different microbial species that coexist together.

These bacteria are not the type that will infect you and cause sickness. These bacteria are the good Samaritans of your body. They help tidy up around the community, keep a neighborhood watch, and contribute to your health in positive ways.

However, they will only treat your body with respect if you maintain a proper habitat. If you behave unhealthily, your internal environment will break down, your bacterial tenants will not be happy, and you will feel sick. But, if you keep a tidy home, your bacteria will happily cooperate with you, and your body will feel great.

Listed below are some examples of how your microbiome controls your internal environment, and this is not even the tip of the iceberg.

1. Your microbiome helps you digest your food so you can absorb more nutrients. It also helps produce essential enzymes, vitamins, and neurotransmitters that the rest of your cells need to function.[9]
2. Good bacteria communicate with your cells to control metabolism, regulate your blood sugar, and control abdominal fat growth.[10]
3. Your good bacteria help fight harmful bacteria by competing for resources and sending signals to activate your immune cells. They also help educate and train your immune cells so your body can fight infections more effectively.[11]
4. Your microbiome helps coordinate wound healing by influencing angiogenesis and stem cell activation.[12]
5. Your gut microbiome is like a second liver because it helps neutralize toxins.[13]
6. Good bacteria help develop and maintain the integrity of your gut lining, which prevents bad stuff from sneaking through your gut wall and causing unwanted inflammation.[14]
7. Your microbiome can modulate gene expression in response to a changing environment in your gut.[15]
8. Your microbiome helps regulate your hormones and can even change the chemistry of your brain. For example, 90% of all serotonin (the feel-good hormone) is produced by gut bacteria.[16] Also, your gut sends nine times more signals to your brain than your brain sends to your gut. The signals from your gut can change the chemistry in your brain and affect your mood, stress, anxiety, hunger, and even your sexual and social behaviors.[17]

If this extensive list does not convince you, consider the fact that the reason you (and every other animal) are alive today is because of a bacterium. The theory reads like this...

A long, long time ago, way before the dinosaurs, the only things that existed were unicellular organisms such as bacteria. Seriously, the only things alive were individual cells that are invisible to the naked eye. There were no plants, no animals, no bugs, and no cavemen, just millions of bacterial cells.

These bacteria survived without oxygen. That was good because, without plants to produce oxygen, the Earth was a very oxygen-less place. Instead, the bacteria survived on hydrogen sulfide that came from volcanoes or thermal vents deep underwater.

Over time, though, the Earth started to get more oxygenated. So, the oxygen-hating bacteria had to find other places to go. One strategy was to hide inside another cell. The bacteria struck a deal with the cell, saying that they would provide energy in return for hospitality. This sounded like a good deal, so the host cell gobbled up the bacterium and let it live inside itself. By making this deal, an entirely new type of organism was born, the eukaryote.

Many years later, the eukaryotes started forming multicellular organisms. Then, those multicellular organisms grew into animals, plants, bugs, and human ancestors.

Every lifeform that you see around you is a multicellular organism. And, in theory, every multicellular organism was born out of this symbiotic relationship.

Your cells still have remnants of the first bacteria that struck such a sweet deal. They are called mitochondria, and they are essential because they provide most of the energy that your cells need to function and survive.

I took some literary liberties with this story, but the moral is that the good bacteria inside you are vitally important for your existence, survival, and health. You depend on your bacteria, and your bacteria depend on you.

Side Note: Major Bacterial Phyla:[18]

Microbiome research is still new, and we still have a lot to learn. However, these are a few common species that everyone should know. You will learn about how to balance these populations in Part III.

Bacterial Family	Individual Species Examples
Firmicutes Family The largest part of the microbiome and the most abundant producer of beneficial fatty acids (short-chain fatty acids - SCFAs) like butyrate Some strains are harmful (e.g., Clostridium difficile causes diarrhea, C. botulinum causes botulism, and C. histolyticum causes gas gangrene)	*L. casei* – found in fermented dairy products and probiotics; protects against food poisoning, diabetes, obesity, cancer, and even depression *L. plantarum* – found in fermented foods and probiotics; produces nutrients like riboflavin and B vitamins *L. reuteri* – found in fermented dairy, sourdough bread, and probiotics; helps produce oxytocin hormone, stimulates angiogenesis, immune-enhancing, and protects against breast and colon tumors *L. rhamnosus* – found in fermented dairy and probiotics; helpful for bacterial overgrowth infections *Ruminococcus* – associated with bean consumption, found in probiotics; produces beneficial SCFAs
Bacteroidetes Family The 2nd largest part of the microbiome, these bacteria also produce lots of SCFAs Some bacteria in this family are pathogenic.	*Bacteroides* – associated with animal-rich diets. They seem to have a neutral impact on health. *Prevotella* – associated with plant-rich diets, produces beneficial SCFAs
Actinobacteria Family Generally beneficial	*Bifidobacterium* – produces SCFAs, found in probiotic supplements
Verrucomicrobia Family These represent a small part of the microbiome, but they are beneficial.	*Akkermansia* – improves blood glucose metabolism, combats obesity, decreases gut inflammation, and protects the walls of your intestines.
Proteobacteria Family In excess, these bacteria may be harmful.	*Desulfovibrionaceae* – harmful due to the production of hydrogen sulfide, which injures gut lining, causing permeability and inflammation

INFLAMMATION & IMMUNE SYSTEM

The function of the immune system is to patrol your body for invaders. Immune cells are constantly patrolling your internal environment as they look for unfriendly organisms. Sometimes, those unfriendly invaders include your own cells that have turned dysfunctional or cancerous. Other times, the organisms are actual invaders coming from the outside world. These bad guys include toxins, chemicals, harmful bacteria, viruses, fungus, molds, etc. For the sake of simplicity, I refer to all these unfriendly organisms as hooligans.[19]

When a hooligan is in your body, it can damage your cells or cause them to malfunction. Your immune system's goal is to prevent these problems from happening. Your body gets rid of the hooligans by kicking them out, destroying them, or stopping them from entering your body in the first place.

To stop the hooligans from entering your body, you use your first line of defense, called your innate immune system. Your innate immune system acts like the walls surrounding a fortress, preventing hooligans from getting into your kingdom.

Like a fortress, any part of your body that is exposed to the outside world will get reinforced with extra protection. For example, your skin has layers of cells stacked on top of each other, thus creating a robust and thick barrier between you and the hooligans. Also, your skin is waterproof so that you can wash off any hooligans that try to hitch a ride. Finally, your skin has a microbiome, which can help defend you against hooligans before they enter your body.

Skin isn't the only part of your body that is exposed to the outside world, though. Your lungs and intestines are, too. Think about it; your digestive tract is just a giant tube running from your mouth to your anus. Anything that enters your mouth and nose (food, water, air, etc.) is coming from the outside world. Every time you breathe, you inhale air from the outside world, as well as all the hooligans floating around with it. Every time you eat, the hooligans on your food come along. Consequently, your digestive and respiratory tracts are loaded with defenses that are similar to your skin fortress.

For example, the cells that line your gut and lungs are held firmly together by tight junctions so that no hooligans can slip through the cracks. Your intestines and lungs are also covered in a layer of mucus that traps hooligans in a sticky goo before they can get into your body. Additionally, your lungs have little hairs (called cilia) that can catch the hooligans and sweep them back upstream. When you exhale or cough, you are expelling some of the hooligans that your cilia have swept away.

Sometimes, though, your fortress can break down. A small scratch is enough to break through your skin barrier and create a hole in your fortress wall. Now hooligans can freely enter your kingdom.

Thankfully, your body prepares for this event. Twenty-four hours a day, your body has watchmen patrolling the gates and looking out for invading hooligans. These watchmen are called white blood cells (WBCs). When your first line of defense fails, your WBCs will flood to the site of damage and start catching hooligans before they can enter your bloodstream.

However, even your WBCs can get overwhelmed by hooligans. If so, your body has another backup plan, called your third line of defense. When your WBCs get overwhelmed, they call in reinforcements by sending a signal to other immune cells, which triggers a process that is much like a game of cops and robbers.

First, your immune cells will grab one of the hooligans and bring it "downtown" (aka to your lymph nodes). At the lymph node, your immune cells will take a picture of the hooligan (like a mugshot).

Your body wants a mugshot because every hooligan has a unique birthmark on its face, called an antigen. When your immune cells take a mugshot of the hooligan, the unique birthmark allows your body to zero in on the hooligan at large.

As soon as they have a mugshot, your immune cells start making millions of copies so they can post the picture around town. These copies are called antibodies, and they get sent through your bloodstream to look for the birthmark that matches their mugshot. Then, when an antibody runs into a hooligan, it latches on like a homing device so your immune cells can find and eliminate the invader.

Your body also keeps some of these mugshots (antibodies) on reserve, like a memory device. If this specific hooligan invades again, you will already have a mugshot on file. Now, you can defend yourself better than before and eliminate the hooligan before it makes you sick.[20]

The critical concept to understand is that almost all these activities constitute a process called **inflammation.** Every time your first line of defense fails, inflammation results. White blood cells flooding to the site of tissue damage, antibodies tagging a hooligan, and any cellular clean-up process can be called inflammation.

You can see inflammation at work when you sprain an ankle. When your ankle gets red, swollen, warm, and tender, you are feeling inflammatory processes in effect. And even though you won't always feel it, the same processes occur in your organs and muscles whenever inflammation is triggered.

But if inflammation is such a powerful healing process, why does our society put so much emphasis on "anti-inflammatory" behaviors? Well, unfortunately, inflammation doesn't just heal damaged tissues; it can also *cause* tissue damage.

Why? Because your body is essentially making a trade-off. It is willing to sacrifice a few healthy cells to protect the whole body from a hooligan invasion. Besides, your body is willing to make this trade-off because inflammation is supposed to be a short-term response. Your body expects to heal an area and then move on, so a small amount of collateral damage is acceptable and quickly dealt with afterward.

But, if the inflammatory response gets out of control, it may persist longer than necessary, and the inflammation can become destructive instead of healing.

Think of inflammation like a cup of coffee. When you have more inflammation than your coffee cup can hold, it will overflow, spill onto your lap, and cause unnecessary damage. If you keep pouring more inflammatory behaviors into the overflowing cup, the unnecessary damage will keep getting worse. Eventually, you could cause damage to entire organs.

If you want to stop the damage (and consequently the symptoms), you need to stop overflowing your cup.

Or you can build a *bigger* cup by following the simple steps in this book.

ANGIOGENESIS

You probably haven't heard of angiogenesis before, but new research shows that angiogenesis can be a valuable self-healing mechanism.

Simply put, angiogenesis is the dimmer switch that controls the growth of tiny blood vessels in your body. And just like inflammation, angiogenesis is all about balance. In order to heal properly, angiogenesis must occur in the right place, at the right time, and in the right amount.

When you have an injury, your body turns on angiogenesis and grows new blood vessels in the damaged area. These new vessels bring extra nutrients and oxygen to your tissues so it can heal faster.[21]

If you've ever peeled off a scab, the skin underneath is pinker than the surrounding skin. This pink color comes from the new blood vessels forming under your scab to heal the cut. That's angiogenesis!

Other times, your body will want to trim back blood vessels; that's *anti*-angiogenesis. Mostly, this process helps prevent the growth of microscopic cancers. By trimming back blood vessels, your body cuts off the supply of oxygen and nutrients so the cancerous cells can't grow. In effect, angiogenesis helps you starve cancer.[22] [23]

CELL REGENERATION

Out with the old, in with the new. Another way that your body heals itself is through a process called cell regeneration. Through this process, your body's old, damaged, or worn-out cells are purposely eliminated so you can usher in a new generation of lively young pups.

Stem cells are what initiate the process of cell regeneration. Stem cells are like shapeshifters that can turn into any cell they want. If your body needs a new liver cell, a stem cell will migrate to the liver, shapeshift into a liver cell, and start making new liver cell babies. If you need a new heart cell, the same stem cell could have shapeshifted into a heart.

Whenever a stem cell travels to an organ, bone, muscle, or tissue, that body part gets a little bit newer. The old cells are recycled, and your new stem cells will regenerate to take their place. Eventually, you will replace all the old cells in an organ with a fresh batch of newborns.

This process occurs much faster than you think. Every 2-4 days, your gut lining completely regenerates. Every 6-12 months, you have a new liver. You have a new layer of skin every month. And even your heart will be renewed after ten years.[24]

In one lifetime, you can replace nearly every cell in your body a few times over. You can literally grow a new body! This is a liberating concept because it means that it is never too late to start rebuilding your health. Every day is a new opportunity for revitalizing your body. Forget about your past because your new cells are built from the actions you take today. If you choose healthy behaviors, your new cells will be stronger and more resilient than the last generation. If you keep practicing unhealthy behaviors, though, the new cells will be just as dysfunctional as the last.

DNA REPAIR & ANTIOXIDATION

Your DNA is always in danger. Inflammation, tobacco, radon, pollution, UV radiation, toxins, stress, pathogens, and even the products of your own cellular metabolism can cause harm to your DNA. In fact, your DNA sustains more than 10,000 damaging effects every day.[25]

But don't worry, this is a natural part of life that you can overcome. Your body knows that damages are inevitable, so it develops elaborate and redundant mechanisms to protect your DNA and promptly repair any errors or injuries.

One way your body protects your DNA is through antioxidants. Antioxidants squelch the toxic byproducts of normal cell function. These byproducts are called reactive oxygen species, or ROS's, and they are like pollutants from your cell factories. By neutralizing the ROS, antioxidants prevent oxidation of your DNA, which helps maintain your cell's longevity.[26]

Another way you can protect your DNA is by taking care of your telomeres. If you think of your DNA as two shoelaces twisted together, telomeres are the plastic aglets on the ends of the lace. Since DNA naturally wears down as you age, your telomeres act as sacrificial endcaps that wear down first before the damage reaches the real DNA. The longer the telomeres, the longer you have until the degradation starts to affect your DNA, and the longer your lifespan.[27]

Once the damage is done, though, antioxidants and telomeres won't be very helpful, so your body repairs your DNA in a few ways.[28] In every cell, you have little repair enzymes that scan DNA to check it for problems. If they recognize a problem, these tiny mechanics will swap, flop, and fill in the cracks of DNA to make it function properly.

Sometimes, though, there is too much damage, and the mechanics don't have time to fix the DNA. If so, your body might try to buy itself more time through the process of epigenetics.

Epigenetics is like a DNA light switch. Throughout life, your environment and your behaviors can cause some genes to turn on and others to turn off. Your DNA turns off by tying itself in a knot. These knots of DNA are called histones.

Other times, your body might want to be more specific. Through a process called methylation, your body can put a small blocker on a particular section of DNA, thus turning that section off. Methylation allows your body to make small, last-minute changes to your DNA just before the replication process begins. Then, when your body is ready, epigenetics can unwind the histone knot or remove the methylation cap to turn DNA back on again.

Through these protection and repair mechanisms, your body prevents your cells from malfunctioning. But, if the DNA damage is too great for your body to repair, it will send the whole cell to the scrapyard and start over again.

DETOXIFICATION & EXCRETION

Everybody poops, pees, sweats, and breathes. Are you doing each of these things at least once per day (besides breathing, of course)?

All these excretion mechanisms are necessary to take the trash out of your body. If you don't take out the trash consistently, the waste will build up, and your cells won't function very well.

Likewise, excretion is good for cleaning up damaged tissue. If a building collapsed and no one cleaned up the rubble, it would be hard to build a new structure in the same space. And if you can't remove damaged cells after an injury, your body won't heal very well, either.

Before excretion occurs, though, the junk must be detoxified. Your main detoxification organ is your liver, which bio-transforms or neutralizes toxins in two phases.

In the first phase, your liver packages the toxic waste and places it on the curb for pick up (aka biotransformation). Phase II consists of picking up the toxic waste from the curb, neutralizing it, and shipping it to the dump. After phase II, some neutralized toxins go back into your blood, and those water-soluble toxins will exit your body as urine or sweat. Meanwhile, other toxins are put in a package of bile, sent to your colon, and excreted as feces.

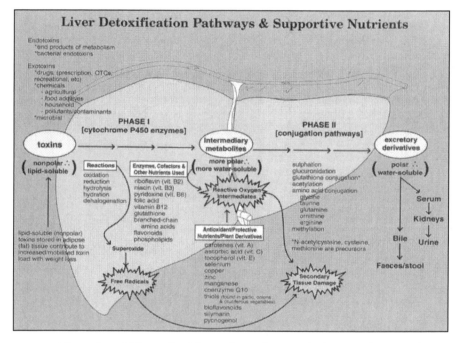

Phase I and Phase II of liver detoxification help transform and neutralize toxins so you can excrete them in your stool, urine, or sweat. Many nutrients are required for these pathways to function correctly.[29]

Sadly, you cannot rely on a '10-day detox cleanse' to solve all your trash removal problems. Detox occurs every day, so you must have a long-term plan if you want lasting results. In part III, you will see that you can adopt a few simple strategies to reduce your toxic load, improve your detox systems, and draw out toxins more effectively.

CHAPTER 8:

STRESS MANAGEMENT

Yuck. Just saying the word 'stress' probably gives you some anxiety. But not all stress is bad. Small amounts of stress can actually help you heal faster. When stress lasts too long, though, it has the reverse effect.

Cortisol is the main offender when it comes to prolonged stress, but that doesn't mean it's always the bad guy. Cortisol acts as a useful pick me up in the morning to get you ready for the day. However, if you are constantly worrying about your endless to-do list or the comment your coworker made last week, your body may be producing too much cortisol at the wrong times. This is happening because your body thinks it needs to prepare for an extended period of physical danger, even if the stress is from a silly argument you had with your friend.

To prepare you for the "physical danger," cortisol will start shutting down different processes in your body. For example, cortisol will slow down the blood supply going to your gut. After all, when you are in real physical danger, your body is more worried about not dying than it is about digesting your last meal. Additionally, excess cortisol will turn off your body's healing and repair mechanisms. Again, your body thinks that all stress is physical stress, so it won't waste energy healing your papercut if it thinks you might be dead soon.

Essentially, when stress lasts too long, the stress-response becomes more damaging than the stressor itself. The excess cortisol dampens digestion, immunity, and all your self-healing mechanisms. And if your stress persists for days or years, your outlook for health doesn't look so great.[30]

Thankfully, with effective stress management strategies (like meditation or spiritual practice), you can "detoxify" your stress and prevent it from persisting for a long time. Therefore, you avoid the damage caused by excess, prolonged cortisol, and you improve your ability to rest, heal, and repair.

PART III
THE SIMPLE STEPS

This is not a diet book.

I repeat, this is not a diet book.

This is a book about lifestyle, about getting the simple things right. It's about forgetting all the noise in the health industry and focusing on the foundations of health.

But don't think of this as a rulebook; think of it as a guidebook. I have cleared many different paths for you, and you get to decide which route to take. Every simple step is taking you in the same direction; they are just alternate paths. Some paths will get you to lifelong youth faster than the others, but the best path is the one you stay on.

Ultimately, I hope you take at least a couple of steps toward creating long-term health. You don't have to tackle all these behaviors at once; take it one step at a time. After all, you may need to change your lifestyle a bit, and that will require a little time, effort, and motivation. Taking on more than you can handle is a recipe for burnout.

To help you on your journey, here are some tips for maximizing success and avoiding burnout:

Tip #1
Start by choosing the behaviors that appeal to you the most.

If a behavior makes you happy *and* it is healthy for you, you should keep doing it. If another behavior seems interesting but difficult to accomplish, lean into the challenge of forming a new and lifelong habit. Even if you fail, the struggle is good for you. If you give something a fighting chance and you still dread it, let it go without worrying; there are plenty of other alternatives.

The most important thing is that you are authentic with yourself and maintain behaviors that add to your happiness. Lifelong Youth is about joy, not suffering.

Tip #2:
There are no magic bullets in health.

Even if you find something that works wonders for you, that does not mean that more is always better. Health is about balance. Too much of a good thing can quickly become detrimental. That's why doctors say that the difference between medicine and poison is dosage. Once you reach a certain threshold, the effect turns negative. So, no matter how good something is for you, don't overdo it. Doing natural things in unnatural amounts is usually unhealthy.

Tip #3
Don't rely on quick fixes.

You cannot build long-term health with quick fixes. Duct tape around a leaky pipe will only last for so long. If you want Lifelong Youth, you're going to have to get down on your hands and knees and thread on some new hardware.

Quick fixes are not all bad, though. Sometimes, your symptoms are just too debilitating to handle. If you can't even think straight because you have a pounding headache, you won't be going for a run anytime soon. If you have a disease that makes your joints hurt, even walking can seem like a chore. Running may help prevent headaches, and walking may reduce joint pain, but I realize how hard it is to make those choices when you're in the throes of agony.

So, the quick fix can help keep your symptoms at bay and enable you to make changes in your life. However, you must know that quick fixes will ONLY help in the short-term; they will not create health in the long run.

P.S. I am not saying you should give up your medications. Always consult with your doctor before doing something like that.

Tip #4
It's okay to splurge sometimes.

I am not here to make you feel bad about eating ice cream, getting 5 hours of sleep, or skipping a workout. Heck, I splurge, too, and it's okay! Being too hard on yourself is not worth it. And the act of stressing about your "bad behavior" may be more damaging than the behavior itself.

All I ask is that you think about why you are splurging and whether you are genuinely making your splurge an enjoyable, rewarding experience. If you are splurging out of boredom, you may want to reconsider.

If your splurge was kind of on accident, that's okay, too. Part of the process of change is failure. Just because you messed up on your "diet" one time doesn't mean you should stop trying altogether. If you splurge one day, treat yourself to some healthy behaviors afterward. When you make healthy choices most of the time, the occasional splurge won't throw you off-track.

Look for the 'Splurge List' addendum in the back of this book. There, you'll find a list of healthy splurge alternatives that still taste like you're getting away with something.

Tip #5:
Habits win championships.

Health is like breaking a giant stone. You will be banging your hammer and chisel 1,000 times over without any noticeable progress. Then on strike 1,001, the stone will finally break. The last strike may have broken the stone, but all the previous strikes are what really mattered.

That is why developing habits is so powerful. Each healthy choice you make is a chink in the stone that gets you closer to a breakthrough. The smallest actions, when performed consistently, have tremendous results.

This is partly because good habits make health come naturally. Once you get into a routine, you won't even have to think about being healthy, and you won't have to rely on self-discipline anymore. You can just live life and let health happen to you as if it were the default option.

Therefore, throughout the book, I will give you some tips and tricks about turning the simple steps into habitual behaviors. Using some ideas from James Clear's 'Atomic Habits,' you won't believe how easy habit formation can be.

STEP #1:

FIND YOUR SENSE OF PURPOSE

Why do you wake up in the morning? If you are like most of the longest-living people on Earth, your reason for getting up is to serve a higher purpose in life.[31] And by having a sense of purpose, some estimates say you could lengthen your life by an average of seven years.[32]

People with a strong sense of purpose are happier, too—your attitude about life changes when you feel like you have a reason for living. Just ask a new parent how they felt when they held their baby in their arms for the first time. Or you can ask the happiest cities in the world because a distinct feature of happy cities is that their citizens have a deep sense of purpose.

In the following pages, I have developed a workbook to help you map your motivations and get re-acquainted with your sense of purpose. Often, we get lost in day-to-day life, and we lose sight of the goals that once defined us. By reconnecting with your sense of purpose, you can get closer to achieving those goals because your actions become more focused, efficient, and productive. This workbook will help you find that sense of purpose again.

As you follow along, write down your answers directly in this book or on a separate sheet of paper. You can also go to lifelongyouthbook.com/resources for a printout.

What are your values?

The words below describe some of the values that are important to people. **Circle** all the values that are **most important to you.** What values do you hold in the highest regard? You may define the words in any way that is meaningful to you, and you may add answers as well.

Abundance	Fairness	Proactivity
Acceptance	Family	Professionalism
Accountability	Flexibility	Punctuality
Achievement	Friendships	Quality
Advancement	Freedom	Recognition
Adventure	Fun	Relationships
Advocacy	Generosity	Reliability
Ambition	Grace	Resilience
Appreciation	Growth	Resourcefulness
Attractiveness	Happiness	Responsibility
Autonomy	Health	Responsiveness
Balance	Honesty	Risk-taking
Being the best	Humility	Safety
Benevolence	Humor	Security
Boldness	Inclusiveness	Service
Brilliance	Independence	Self-Control
Calmness	Individuality	Selflessness
Caring	Innovation	Simplicity
Challenge	Inspiration	Spirituality
Charity	Intelligence	Stability
Cheerfulness	Intuition	Success
Cleverness	Joy	Teamwork
Community	Kindness	Thankfulness
Commitment	Knowledge	Thoughtfulness
Compassion	Leadership	Traditionalism
Cooperation	Learning	Trustworthiness
Collaboration	Love	Understanding
Consistency	Loyalty	Uniqueness
Contribution	Making a difference	Usefulness
Creativity	Mindfulness	Versatility
Credibility	Motivation	Vision
Curiosity	Optimism	Warmth
Daring	Open-Mindedness	Wealth
Decisiveness	Originality	Well-Being
Dedication	Passion	Wisdom
Dependability	Peace	Zeal
Diversity	Perfection	_____
Empathy	Performance	_____
Encouragement	Personal development	_____
Enthusiasm	Playfulness	_____
Ethics	Popularity	_____
Excellence	Power	
Expressiveness	Preparedness	

Of the values that you circled, choose your top 10, and rank them in order of importance (1 = most important).

1. _____   5. _____   9. _____

2. _____   6. _____   10. _____

3. _____   7. _____

4. _____   8. _____

Why is your #1 value so important to you? How did you develop this value?

_____

_____

Using the same 10 values, which values do you live up to the most? For example, a college student may value loyalty as #1 and learning as #10. However, the student might spend most of her time studying and often neglect her commitments. Below, the student would put studying/learning at #1, whereas loyalty might rank as #5. These values might be challenging to quantify but give it your best guess.

1. _____   5. _____   9. _____

2. _____   6. _____   10. _____

3. _____   7. _____

4. _____   8. _____

Are both your lists in roughly the same order, or are there discrepancies? In other words, are you living up to your values in the same way that you prioritize your values? How might you explain what happened? Has your behavior changed compared to the past? What is different? How have your circumstances changed? Answer whichever question you like.

_____

_____

_____

Did you notice any discrepancies between your values and your behaviors? If so, think about what might happen if you don't change your behaviors at all. What is the worst thing that could happen if you let things continue as is? This is not a sarcastic question. Honestly, how bad could things get if you don't change anything?

_____

_____

_____

How might you change your behaviors so that you will live up to the values you hold in the highest regard? What would you like to do differently to realign your actions with your values?

_____

_____

_____

If you make these changes to your behaviors, what is the best outcome that you can imagine happening?

_____

_____

_____

-     -   -

It is okay if none of the values that you listed were related to health or longevity. However, since you are reading this book, we are kind of obligated to talk about health. So, what are at least three reasons why you care about health? In other words, why are you reading this book?

1._____

2._____

3._____

People usually want to be healthy because they have a more profound goal in mind. They either want to achieve something, or they want to continue doing the things they currently enjoy. What are your goals, and when do you want to achieve them? Five years from now? 20 years from now? Maintain it forever?

Goal #1:	Goal #2:	Goal #3:
Achieved by:	Achieved by:	Achieved by:

Now, let's see if you feel ready for change. On the right, rate how important it is for you to start making healthier choices in your life? 1 means 'not important at all' and 10 means 'most important.'

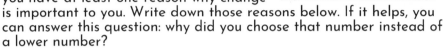

If you chose a number greater than 1, you have at least one reason why change is important to you. Write down those reasons below. If it helps, you can answer this question: why did you choose that number instead of a lower number?

_____

_____

_____

Now, do the same thing for your confidence. Rate how confident you are that you can make the changes necessary to live a healthier and more youthful life. 1 means 'not confident at all' and 10 means 'extremely confident.'

If you chose a number greater than 1, you have at least some confidence in yourself. That's great! Write down some reasons why you have confidence in your abilities. For example, maybe you accomplished other changes in the past, which gives you confidence that you can make changes in your health behaviors.

_____

_____

_____

Rate your readiness to change. Do you feel ready to act? 1 means 'not ready at all' and 10 means 'extremely ready, and you have already started making changes.'

If you chose a number greater than 1, you are ready. You may not be "all in" yet, but you are willing to take some sort of action. If you want, you can write down some reasons why you are ready, but any amount of readiness is all you need.

_____

_____

_____

For each goal that you listed on the other page, write down your answers to these questions:

- What is the best possible outcome that could happen if you achieved this goal?
- If you didn't change a thing, how soon would you achieve this goal? Would you achieve it at all?
- What is the worst possible outcome if you failed to achieve this goal?

	Goal #1	Goal #2	Goal #3
The best possible outcome that you are hoping for			
Status quo, how things are right now			
The worst possible outcome if you fail			

Once you've completed the table, look at your answers again. But, this time, have this question in mind: why do you *need* to change? (Most likely, your answer will be "to avoid the bad outcomes and to achieve the good outcomes.")

After you've thought of why you **need** to change, give me some reasons why you **want** to change? Give your 3 best reasons.

1._____

2. _____

3. _____

How do you hope this book might help you? What do you think we can accomplish together?

_____

_____

Now, summarize your answers in the table below. You can add new answers, too. This is kind of like a pro-con chart but with a twist.

Advantages of NOT changing	Disadvantages of changing
Disadvantages of NOT changing	Advantages of changing

Well done! Now, let's make a plan.

First, list five healthy behaviors that you would enjoy doing. Maybe you like playing sports, or maybe you are more of a chef and enjoy cooking healthy food.

1._____

2._____

3._____

4._____

5._____

Who do you want on your team? Which people could be helpful or supportive on your road to Lifelong Youth? Friend power is more potent than willpower, so having a friend or family member as a health coach can help keep you accountable and motivated. Even if your support system is on a social network, it still counts.

What impediments or obstacles might you encounter along the way?

Obstacle #1:	Obstacle #2:	Obstacle #3:

How might you overcome those obstacles?

Obstacle #1	Obstacle #2	Obstacle #3

How will you know if your plan is working? What are some markers for health that you can use to guide you? Here are some examples that might stimulate your creativity:

Weight

Blood test biomarkers (e.g., Hemoglobin A1C, C-reactive protein, Homocysteine, Complete blood count, Lipid profile, Waist:Hip ratio, Heart rate variability)

Daily energy levels

Fitness goals (mile time, total walking distance, lifting PR)

Number of days off work due to sickness

_____

_____

_____

What gives you confidence that you can do this?

_____

Are you going to do it?

_____

When do you think you'll start?

_____

Now, let's summarize your work. Look back on your previous answers and fill them in below. You can hang this summary page on your fridge, bathroom mirror, or somewhere you can see it every morning.

Goal #1:	Goal #2:	Goal #3:
Disadvantages of NOT changing		Advantages of changing

5 healthy behaviors that I'd enjoy doing.

Step #1 _____

Step #2 _____

Step #3 _____

Step #4 _____

Step #5 _____

Who is on my team? Who can help support me?_____

_____

Obstacle #1:	Obstacle #2:	Obstacle #3:
What will I do when I encounter this obstacle?	What will I do when I encounter this obstacle?	What will I do when I encounter this obstacle?

I will know it is working if... (blood tests, fitness goals, energy levels, sick days, etc.)

_____

Statement of readiness:

I am confident, ready, and prepared to make a change. I know
that every day is another opportunity for health because I have new
cells that want to be as healthy as possible. I know there will be
obstacles, and I know how to overcome them. Even if I falter, I know
how to bounce back. I have people that I can lean on for support,
and I have ways to track my success. I can do this!

Signed,

_____

Bonus: The Centenarian Olympics[33]

Most people think that all 100-year-olds are frail and immobile, but that is not the case. In Dan Buettner's book, _The Blue Zones_[34], the centenarians he studied were still active, and some were still working!

So, for this exercise, imagine being an active 100-year-old. What activities of daily life would you like to do?

Remember, you have no serious illnesses, and you are by no means about to keel over, but you are not the 20-year-old you once were. You'd be surprised what a 100-year-old can do but keep it within reason.

Here are some suggestions that may help you get started. If they resonate with you, feel free to use them for your own Centenarian Olympic goals.

- Carry 2-4 bags of groceries from the car to the house, or walk to and from the grocery store (strength/endurance)
- Get in and out of a car without pulling on the doorframe (strength)
- Climb 4 flights of stairs without feeling out of breath (endurance)
- Get up and down off the floor by yourself (agility)
- Lift 30lbs overhead (strength)
- Be able to stand on wobbly, bouncy busses or trains (balance)
- Fly in an airplane (social)
- Walk 2-5 miles on an uneven trail (endurance)
- Be able to squat or lunge in the garden (agility)
- Run (even if it is slow) for any distance - 20ft still counts (strength)
- Jump off a diving board and swim to the wall (strength/balance)
- Push/Pull open a heavy door (strength/balance)
- Read every day (mental)
- Be able to perform a difficult brain game like a crossword or sudoku puzzle (mental)
- Have the dexterity and skill to draw or paint (social/mental)
- Cook your own meals every day (social/emotional)
- Visit family and be able to play on the ground with your great grandkids (social)
- Carry on a long conversation with your friends or family (social/mental)
- Maintain your memories and be able to tell stories of your life (mental)
- Feel energized throughout the day without napping (mental/energy)
- Maintain all your senses - especially smell, vision, and hearing (mental)
- Be fully aware of your surroundings (mental)

How about you? What are 5-10 activities that you want to do when you are 100 years old? Think mostly in terms of movement, cognition, and emotional/social health.

1. _____
2. _____
3. _____
4. _____
5. _____
6. _____
7. _____
8. _____
9. _____
10. _____

How about at age 90, 80, 70, or 60? Work backward until you reach your current age. With each decade, your goals will probably become more ambitious. When you get to your current age, write down the goals that you have for yourself. What must you be able to do 1-3 years from now if you expect to meet your 100-year-old goals?

1. _____
2. _____
3. _____
4. _____
5. _____

Have you met the goals that you expect from a person your age?

_____
_____
_____

If not, what are you going to do about it? Consider going back to the beginning of this chapter. Then, use these as your new goals in the 'Find Your Sense of Purpose' workbook.

Step #2

Eat, Papa, Eat!

"If diet is wrong, medicine is of no use. If diet is right, medicine is of no need."
- Ayurvedic proverb

These days, people only talk about diet when they want to lose weight or heal an ailment. They think diet is a short term, quick fix for their health concerns. So, in honor of that, I will say again that THIS IS NOT A DIET BOOK.

Instead of telling you what to eat and when to eat it, I will simply show you a world of amazing foods that are delicious, affordable, and healthful. Then, you get to decide what foods you want to eat from that list.

And, thankfully, you don't have to be perfect. If you eat these foods *most* of the time (like 80% of the time), you can get away with misbehaving every once in a while.

EXAMPLE

For the rest of Step #2 (and the rest of this book), I will be using the following table to help summarize the information. Along the X-axis is a list of your body's self-regulating and self-healing systems (which we discussed in Part II). Along the Y-axis will be a list of different foods or behaviors. If a behavior or food has a positive impact on one of your self-healing or self-regulating systems, you'll see a checkmark in the associated column. Then, the bullet points below the chart will describe some examples of that effect.

	Self-Regulation	Structure & Mobility	Microbiome	Immune Balance	Angiogenic Balance	DNA Repair & Antioxidants	Regeneration & Autophagy	Detox & Excretion	Stress Mgmt.
Subcategory									
Subcategory									

✔ = the behavior is beneficial to the associated healing system
✘ = the behavior is potentially harmful to the associated healing system

 Examples of the food/behavior's self-regulation benefits.

 Examples of the food/behavior's structure & mobility benefits.

 Examples of the food/behavior's microbiome benefits.

 Examples of the food/behavior's immune system benefits.

 Examples of the food/behavior's angiogenic benefits.

 Examples of the food/behavior's DNA protection benefits.

 Examples of the food/behavior's cell regeneration benefits.

 Examples of the food/behavior's detox & excretion benefits.

 Examples of the food/behavior's stress management benefits.

This book would be 1000 pages long if I listed every benefit associated with a food or behavior. So, the bullet points below the table will focus on the most essential, unique, or exciting effects. For example, I'm not going to discuss every vitamin and mineral that makes a carrot healthy for you. Instead, I'll simply summarize the main ideas. If you want more detailed information, you can check out the resources section listed in the appendix.

VEGETABLES, TUBERS, & ROOTS

First, the veggies. Since it would take far too long to talk about all the different types of vegetables, I have separated them into various categories. Keep in mind that this chart is a summary, and not all the vegetables in each group will have the same effects on your self-healing systems. However, you can see that vegetables are a great way to start your health journey because they check almost every box.

Best of the best: leafy greens (kale, spinach, etc.), broccoli, brussels sprouts, pepper[35]

	SELF-REGULATION	STRUCTURE & MOBILITY	MICROBIOME	IMMUNE BALANCE	ANGIOGENIC BALANCE	DNA REPAIR & ANTIOXIDANTS	REGENERATION & AUTOPHAGY	DETOX & EXCRETION	STRESS MGMT.
LEAFY GREEN VEGETABLES*	✓	✓	✓	✓	✓	✓	✓	✓	
CRUCIFEROUS VEGETABLES*	✓	✓	✓	✓	✓	✓	✓	✓	
COLORFUL VEGETABLES*	✓	✓	✓	✓	✓	✓	✓	✓	
HERBS & SPICES	✓	✓	✓	✓	✓	✓	✓	✓	✓

✓ = the food is beneficial to the associated healing system

*Leafy Green Vegetables = kale, spinach, green/red leaf lettuce, dandelion, collard greens, beet leaves, swiss chard
*Cruciferous Vegetables = broccoli, cauliflower, brussels sprouts, arugula, bok choy, cabbage, kohlrabi, radish, turnip
*Colorful Vegetables = pepper, carrot, beet, sweet potato, squash, Chinese celery, fiddleheads (baby ferns)

- Vegetables are packed with vitamins and minerals, so they are an efficient way to get lots of nutrients without many calories.

- Beets, rosemary, pepper, Chinese celery, and other vegetables help improve blood flow, especially in your brain.[36] [37]

- Eating leafy green vegetables helps slow the aging process of your brain. One study showed that people who eat just one cup of leafy greens per day had a brain that acted 11 years younger.[38]

- Vegetables feed your muscles and help maintain bone calcium.[39]

- Your gut bacteria love eating fiber-rich vegetables. And when they do, they produce a fatty acid called butyrate. Butyrate is responsible for giving you more energy, improving your brain and liver function, and helping you build a healthy gut lining. Plus, butyrate is anti-inflammatory and has anti-obesity, anti-diabetes, and anti-cancer properties.[40] Eating fiber also results in the production of propionate and acetate. Propionate helps lower cholesterol, reduces inflammation, and improves digestive health. Acetate keeps you from feeling hungry by stimulating the release of the satiety hormone called leptin.[41]

    Examples of fiber-rich vegetables: tubers, roots, yams, jicama, rutabagas, parsnips, sweet potatoes, taro root, cassava, Yucca, artichoke, chicory, radicchio, Belgian endive, leek, and okra

- Vegetables that contain inulin stimulate *Akkermansia municiphilia*. This bacterium produces mucus that protects your gut wall, activates your immune system, and lowers blood glucose.[42] [43]

    Examples of inulin rich veggies: chicory, Belgian endive, radicchio, escarole, artichoke, sugar beet, plantain, onion, garlic, dandelion root, and jicama. Wheat is a significant source of inulin, so if you decide to go gluten-free, add these other inulin-rich foods to your repertoire.

- Brassica foods (like broccoli, cauliflower, bok choy, cabbage, kale, rutabaga, turnip, and arugula) help decrease harmful bacteria populations via antimicrobial peptides (AMPs).[44]

- Most vegetables prevent excess inflammation and enhance immune function.[45] Aged garlic and broccoli sprouts, for example, increase your immune system's abundance of T cells and natural killer cells, thus making a more effective company of hooligan-killers. [46] [47] [48]

- Herbs and spices are wonderful immune enhancers. For example, chile peppers increase your circulating white blood cells and B cells (via capsaicin).[49] Licorice root activates T and B cell production.[50] And curcumin (the compound found in turmeric spice) is one of the few known substances that can reduce brain inflammation.[51]

Yellow-orange vegetables are great for eye health because the compound, Zeaxanthin, accumulates in the retina to protect the blood vessels in the eye.[52]

> *Examples of Zeaxanthin-rich vegetables: Corn, saffron, kale, mustard greens, spinach, watercress, collard greens, and swiss chard.*

Brassica foods (containing brassinin and sulforaphane) help you stop cancerous growths with their antiangiogenic properties.[53]

> *Examples of brassica-rich foods: broccoli, cauliflower, bok choy, cabbage, kale, rutabaga, turnip, arugula.*

These spices help modulate angiogenic balance: ginseng, rosemary, peppermint, oregano, turmeric, licorice, and cinnamon.[54] [55] [56] [57] [58]

Cruciferous vegetables (like broccoli, cauliflower, and brussels sprouts) can reduce the activity of 36 genes associated with colon cancers.[59]

Turmeric/curcumin spice activates tumor suppressor genes to help protect you from cancer.[60]

Many vegetables contain protective antioxidants like vitamins A, C, E, and selenium. Meanwhile, red pepper, broccoli, and Brussels sprouts contain high cysteine, a precursor for glutathione, your most potent antioxidant.

Most vegetables help protect your stem cells from oxidative damage. This may result in better digestion, improved fitness, better sexual experiences, and faster healing.

Yellow-orange veggies (containing Zeaxanthin) improve stem cell performance,[61] which may help your organs regenerate more efficiently, so you can stay healthier for longer.

Turmeric/curcumin spice increases the number of circulating stem cells, thereby improving your healing powers.[62]

Vegetables upregulate phase II of your liver's detoxification pathway through nutrients like alpha-carotene, beta-carotene, quercetin, chrysin, luteolin, D-glucaric-acid, cysteine, and folate.[63]

Sulfur-rich vegetables contain metallothionein, which chelates/binds metal and other toxins. Cilantro is also a chelator. It binds to metals like mercury and lead.[64]

Certain herbs and foods are called adaptogens because they help you adapt to stress. Interestingly, most adaptogens come from plants that have extensive root systems. Some examples are Asian ginseng, Ashwagandha, Aacope, and Rhodiola.

Habit Hacks:

- Habit formation starts with your sense of identity. Instead of saying, "I need to eat more vegetables," say to yourself, "I am the type of person who eats healthy now, and healthy people eat more vegetables."
- Make vegetables obvious and visible in your fridge. You are more likely to grab a healthy snack when it is the closest thing in reach.
- Consider writing down this new habit: "When I grab a snack from the fridge/cupboard, I will also grab a vegetable. I have to eat the vegetable first, and if I'm still hungry, I can have the other snack." This habit forces you to nail down a specific time and location where the healthy behavior will occur. You are also stacking the vegetable-eating habit on top of an existing habit (grabbing a snack). Thirdly, by having a snack, you reward yourself after completing the vegetable-eating habit.

Tips & Tricks:

- Eat raw vegetables as often as you can, but feel free to bake, fry, boil, and steam your veggies, too. While it is true that cooking results in some nutrient loss, cooked veggies are still a much healthier choice than most mealtime alternatives.
- Vegetable dip is okay if it gets you to eat more raw vegetables. Of course, some dips are better than others, but I'm a sucker for Ranch, too. Just start each vegetable escapade with a non-dipped veggie and see how you feel. Or try peanut butter on your vegetables. Seriously, just try it.
- Eat the entirety of the vegetable if you can. The stems of broccoli, mushrooms, kale, and other plants are usually the healthiest part.
- Choose smoothies over juices. Juiced vegetables lack one of the main ingredients that make plants healthy, the fiber! Smoothies, though, retain all the healthy fiber. Also, store-bought vegetable juices have hidden junk like artificial sweeteners and additives.
- People like to vilify starchy vegetables due to their high-carb, glucose-spiking effects. I say, don't beat yourself up about this. If you add healthy fats to your starches (like coconut oil or extra virgin olive oil), you will lower the glucose spike. Potatoes, for example, are very starchy, but adding healthy fats will reduce the glycemic index. Also, if you cool the potato and reheat it later, the starches turn into resistant starches, which are healthy fuel for your microbiome. The more times you heat and cool a potato, the more resistant starches will form. In effect, the once-vilified potato becomes a superfood for your good bacteria. Plus, if your choice is between a starchy vegetable and a fast food or microwave meal, the starchy vegetable should always win.

- As Michael Pollan would say, "Eat food. Not too much. Mostly plants."[65] My addition is, "Eat food that you cook yourself, and if you can, plant a garden."
- Check out imperfectproduce.com to get fresh and cheap produce delivered to your door. The veggies from Imperfect Produce may be ugly, but that's why you get such a good deal!
- The Environmental Working Group has some great resources to help you choose organic foods. Some plants are very susceptible to pesticide accumulation, so the EWG puts these in the "Dirty Dozen" list. Other plants are relatively resilient, though, so you don't need to worry so much about buying the organic version; these are called the "Clean Fifteen." Check them out by visiting the websites below.
  https://www.ewg.org/foodnews/dirty-dozen.php;
  https://www.ewg.org/foodnews/clean-fifteen.php;
  https://www.ewg.org/foodnews/summary.php

Side Note: Vegetarian & Veganism

I was a vegetarian for five years, so I understand the sentiments of abstaining from meat. However, if you are considering vegetarianism, you must be more strategic with your diet to optimize your nutritional content. For example, you will likely need to supplement with EPA and DHA fatty acids if you are not eating fish or algae. Plants contain a lot of omega-3 fats called alpha-linoleic acid (ALA). However, only ~5% of dietary ALA gets converted into EPA or DHA.[66] Consequently, vegetarians may risk having an unhealthy ratio of omega-6 to omega-3 fats, leading to excess inflammation in the body.

Also, grains and legumes (such as soy) are often a staple in vegetarian diets. These foods, though, contain antinutrients (phytates, lectins, and trypsin inhibitors), which are known to reduce the absorption of various minerals like iron, calcium, and magnesium. Soaking beans and grains in water for 24hrs before cooking them may reduce this anti-nutrient effect.[67] Fermentation also reduces anti-nutrient qualities (e.g., Tempeh, fermented soy).[68]

Finally, your gut cannot absorb vitamin B-12 from plant sources very well. If you are concerned about B-12 deficiency, you can supplement with methyl B-12 under the tongue or use liberal amounts of nutritional yeast in your cooking. Animal products are the best source of B-12, so if you are willing to eat some animals, organ meats (liver) and shellfish will get you the most bang for your buck.

FRUIT

Again, it would take far too long to talk about all the different types of fruits, so I have created various categories. The fruits within each group have similar effects on your self-healing systems but in varying amounts.

Best of the best: berries (blueberry, raspberry, mulberry), avocado, cacao (>80% dark chocolate), olives, green banana, crispy pear

	Self-Regulation	Structure & Mobility	Microbiome	Immune Balance	Angiogenic Balance	DNA Repair & Antioxidants	Regeneration & Autophagy	Detox & Excretion	Stress Mgmt.
Berries	✓		✓	✓	✓	✓	✓	✓	
Stone Fruit*	✓				✓	✓	✓	✓	✓
Citrus Fruit*	✓	✓	✓	✓		✓		✓	
Other Fruit*	✓	✓	✓	✓	✓	✓	✓	✓	

✓ = the food is beneficial to the associated healing system

*Stone Fruit = peach, plum, nectarine, lychee, apricot, cherry, coconut
*Citrus Fruit = grapefruit, orange, guava, kiwifruit, pineapple, lemon, papaya, lime, kumquat, ugli fruit, buddha's hand
*Other Fruit = tomato, avocado, cacao (80% dark chocolate), pomegranate, apple, eggplant, cantaloupe, fig (technically a flower)

All fruits have healthy vitamins and minerals that are crucial for cellular metabolism and function. Without them, you'll die much sooner than you might like.

Dark chocolate boosts brain function and enhances memory.[69]

Fruits with high vitamin C help make collagen, so you'll have stronger tendons, fascia, and ligaments to prevent you from getting injured.
> *Examples of vitamin C-rich fruits: Cherry tomatoes, grapefruit, guava, oranges, strawberries, grapes, cacao (>80% dark chocolate).*

Five prunes per day may prevent bone loss in postmenopausal women.[70]

Fruits that are high in polyphenols support microbiome balance. Berries are the same color on the outside as they are on the inside, which signifies their polyphenol richness.[71]

Fig (technically a flower, not a fruit) and kiwifruit are full of prebiotic fibers that feed your microbiome.[72]

Dark chocolate helps balance your microbiome and feeds the bacterial species called *Bifidobacterium* and *Lactobacilli.*[73]

Pomegranate, cranberry, and concord grape juice increase *Akkermansia municiphilia* populations, thus combating gut inflammation and obesity. These bugs also improve your immune function and strengthen the protective mucous layer in your gut.[74][75]

Black raspberry, blackberry, and pomegranate have ellagic acid to improve your immune system's ability to detect and destroy cancer cells.[76]

High-vitamin C fruits increase the production of T regulatory cells, which restores immune balance and turns down inflammation.[77]

Blueberries help calm-down excess inflammation by deactivating your immune cells (like myeloid dendritic cells and natural killer cells).[78][79]

Cranberries and apples balance both sides of angiogenesis (via quercetin, and ursolic acid) while also inhibiting inflammation.[80][81] Berries are great at this, too, especially blueberries.[82] Fruit skins contain ursolic acid, so don't peel your apples before eating them.

Tomatoes are antiangiogenic due to lycopene, rutin, and beta-cryptoxanthin. They are especially impressive at combating prostate cancer.[83]

Stone fruit like peaches, plums, nectarines, apricots, cherries, mango, and lychee inhibit blood vessel growth (antiangiogenic). Plums and cherries are the best at this.[84] Dark chocolate is antiangiogenic, too.[85]

Lycopene protects against UV radiation. Eat or drink the following fruits before getting exposed to the sun, X-rays, or airplane radiation: tomato, watermelon, guava, and grapefruit.[86] These fruits are also protective against DNA damage that can be caused by an infection.[87]

Kiwifruit improves antioxidant function and helps you repair your DNA more quickly (via vitamin C, chlorogenic acid, and quinic acid).[88]

Black raspberry, blackberry, and pomegranate (due to ellagic acid, anthocyanin, & quercetin) are stem cell activators that also help improve your blood vessel flexibility.[89] [90]

Cocoa is a stem cell activator due to the flavanols, which also improve blood circulation.[91]

Grapes and red wine activate the cardiac stem cells that usually lie dormant in your heart.[92] This is primarily due to resveratrol, which is also found in cranberries, blueberries, peanuts, and pistachios. These effects were only seen in high doses, though, so you might consider taking supplemental resveratrol.

Foods with chlorogenic acid (e.g., blueberries, stone fruits, and eggplant) improve stem cell survival by making them more resilient to stress. Meanwhile, they help kill cancerous stem cells.[93]

Mango (via the compound mangiferin) is antitumor and antidiabetic because it helps regenerate your pancreas' beta cells. It may also regenerate bones.[94] [95] [96] [97]

Dark chocolate has lots of vitamin C, which is a potent antioxidant.[98]

Berries are also well-known for being loaded with antioxidants.[99] Blueberries are the best.

The following fruits are good at promoting phase II of liver detoxification: citrus fruits, apples, cherries, apricots, bananas, and peaches.[100]

Dark chocolate ingestion is associated with reduced stress markers like cortisol and adrenaline.[101]

Habits Hacks:

- Decide who you want to be. Do you want to be a healthy person? If so, then what would a healthy person do? Do healthy people enjoy eating fruit? Yes, and so will you because you are a healthy person.

- Make fruit visible. Put a fruit bowl in a prominent location, so it is easy to grab on your way out the door. Choosing fruit as your midday snack will always be a better choice than whatever is in the vending machine. Similarly, don't leave junk in the house. If junk is easy to get, you'll undoubtedly eat it. But if all your cravings require a special drive to the grocery store, you are more likely to choose the healthier option in your immediate vicinity.

- Use temptation to your advantage. If you are craving a treat, serve up a dish with half as much treat as usual and occupy the other half with fresh or frozen fruit.

- Write down your habit. For example, after dinner, tell yourself that you will eat fruit for dessert at least one day per week.

Tips & Tricks:

- Dried fruit is a good splurge food compared to some other snack options, but don't splurge so hard that you end up at the bottom of a bag in one sitting. It is easy to eat a lot of dried fruit because it isn't as dense as whole fruit. But eating more dried fruit means you will get a more concentrated dose of sugar.

- Like I said in the vegetable section, smoothies are much better than juices. Juiced fruit lacks fiber, while a smoothie still contains all the benefits of the whole fruit. Also, when you make fruit into juice, your body absorbs the sugar very quickly, which causes a spike in your blood sugar. Smoothies cause a blood sugar jump, too, but not as drastic as juices. If you can sneak some vegetables into your smoothie, that is even better.

- Eat the entire fruit, including the stem. Often, the stem or leaves are the most nutrient-dense (e.g., the leaves on a strawberry).

- Put dark chocolate under your tongue until it melts away. You'll notice that after a few pieces of chocolate, your craving will be satisfied.

- Again, check out these resources from the Environmental Working Group about organic versus nonorganic foods:
https://www.ewg.org/foodnews/dirty-dozen.php;
https://www.ewg.org/foodnews/clean-fifteen.php;
https://www.ewg.org/foodnews/summary.php

PRODUCTS FROM HEALTHY ANIMALS

If you're going to eat an animal, would you rather eat a sick animal or a healthy one?

Well, here's some bad news, most of America's farm animals are unhealthy. Large-scale farms are more interested in quantity instead of quality, so they take shortcuts that jeopardize the health of our livestock. We feed livestock unnatural diets like corn, bread, candy, and hormones because it fattens the animal faster. Then, to mask the unhealthiness, farmers will pump the animal with antibiotics and medicines (because diseased meat isn't very profitable).

Now, all those antibiotics, hormones, and inflammatory markers from the unnatural diet are coursing through the animal's body. When you eat meat or drink milk from that animal, all that junk is now causing havoc in your own body.

So, if you want to get health benefits from the animals you eat, the animals themselves must be healthy, too. When the animal is unhealthy, its nutritional content is overshadowed by the adverse effects of inflammation, antibiotics, and unhealthy living conditions.

When buying animal products, try to make sure the animal was raised humanely. Most of the time, you will only get this information by talking to local farmers, but here are some basic rules to help you decide if the animal lived a healthy life.

- Cows: pasture-raised, grazing on prairie grasses (aka grass-fed and grass-finished)
- Chickens: free to peck at grubs, insects, and food scraps (>8ft² of land per bird)
- Goats: free to graze on grasses, twigs, leaves, and food scraps

Best of the best: wild game, organ meat (liver), bone broth, free-range chicken eggs, duck eggs, milk/cheese/butter from grass-fed cows

Products from Healthy Animals

	Self-Regulation	Structure & Mobility	Microbiome	Immune Balance	Angiogenic Balance	DNA Repair & Antioxidants	Regeneration & Autophagy	Detox & Excretion	Stress Mgmt.
Muscle Meat	✓	✓			✓	✓		✓	
Organ Meat/Offal	✓	✓						✓	
Eggs	✓	✓		✓				✓	
Milk, Cheese, or Butter	✓	✓	✓		✓			✓	

✓ = the food is beneficial to the associated healing system

- Most animal products have a complete amino acid profile, which means you get all your essential amino acids at once. Not all the proteins get absorbed, though. The amount of protein that you absorb from food is called the biological value. Chicken and cow meat have a biological value of about 80, which means 80% of the protein is absorbed. Cow's milk has a biological value of 91.[102] Eggs have the highest biological value of all, at 97%![103]

- The purpose of the egg and egg yolk is to provide the developing baby chicken with all the required proteins, fats, cholesterol, vitamins, minerals, and growth factors that it needs. When you eat an egg, you get all those excellent nutrients, too, which help you build robust and high-functioning cells.

- Animals that eat grass have more vitamins than grain-fed animals (e.g., beta carotene, folic acid, K2, and vitamin E).[104] Also, the ratio of omega-3 to omega-6 fats in grass-fed products is closer to the ideal ratio of 1:1, while grain-fed cow products have a ratio closer to 14:1.

Animal meats (especially organ meat) benefit your bones, muscles, and joints because they are rich in collagen and protein.

Milk builds strong bones, but not on its own. For the calcium in milk to enter your bones, you need to be exercising. If you don't exercise, your bones won't feel pressured to get stronger, so they won't absorb as much calcium.

Yogurt (with no added junk) is both probiotic & prebiotic.[105]

Cheese made from raw milk is highly probiotic. However, US-made cheeses are less beneficial because we pasteurize our milk.[106] Some examples of great European cheeses include Parmigiano-Reggiano, Gouda, & Camembert.

Eggs contain substances to help protect you against bacterial and viral infections. For instance, they help prevent pathogens from clinging on to your cells.[107] [108]

Chicken soup (from healthy chickens) decreases inflammation and thus improves immunity.[109]

Dark chicken meat (like chicken thighs) has more vitamin K2 than white meat (like chicken breast) and provides more antiangiogenic benefits.[110] K2 also helps coagulate a wound and mineralize bone. Then, when you're done healing your injuries, K2 can help dissolve the clot so it doesn't clog up your arteries.[111] [112]

Cheese may contain vitamin K2 as well. Some great cheeses with K2 include Muenster, Gouda, Camembert, Edam, Stilton, & Emmental.

Eating healthy red meat 1-2 times per day is associated with longer telomere length.[113] [114]

Eggs have some antioxidant properties and contain detoxification nutrients such as sulfur, folate, cysteine, and B12.

Most animal products (especially organ meats like liver) are rich in folate and B12, which help you methylate or neutralize toxins.

Yogurts, cheeses, milk, and butter contain cysteine, a precursor for your most potent antioxidant, called glutathione.

Veal, chicken, beef, turkey, and some milk products contain sulfur, which helps with phase II of liver detoxification.

Things to consider regarding meat consumption:

Humans cannot grow crops in many areas of the world because the landscape is too rocky or steep. However, animals are often able to graze on this land. Raising livestock, then, might be necessary if we want to feed the world. Crops, alone, may not be able to.

Even though raising livestock is often vilified as bad for the environment, it does not have to be. We know how to raise livestock in a highly productive yet sustainable and regenerative way. Unfortunately, products from regenerative farms tend to have a higher price tag than their corn-fed, industrially raised counterparts. This is misleading, though, because the actual cost of industrial animal products is much higher than the price tag.

For example, corn is a water-hungry crop. It has been shown that industrial farming often results in wasted water, soil depletion, and environmental degradation. However, these costly effects are not factored into the price of corn-fed cows because we artificially reduce the price of factory-farmed meat products through subsidies and grants. When you factor in farmer subsidies, land value, water usage, shipping costs, processing costs, and healthcare expenses (for both the humans and the livestock), the cost of that corn-fed animal product goes way up. Conversely, when you buy healthy and locally sourced animal products, almost all the costs are factored into the price. The price tag and the real cost of healthy animals are basically equal.

So, the next time you reach for the "cheaper" meat option, consider the real cost of that food, not just the price tag. Paying a higher price for meat will reduce your consumption (which may be healthier for you), and it tells the world that you prefer healthy animals over cheap animals. As a result, healthy animals may become more affordable.

The most compelling argument against eating meat is that it stimulates your mTOR gene. When mTOR activates, it tells your cells to stay in a state of growth and reproduction. This state is okay when you are growing or healing, but it's not so great for longevity because you end up wasting a lot of energy for no good reason. Your body wants to conserve energy, and constantly stepping on the mTOR gas pedal is taxing on your system. As a result, your body will likely wear out more quickly.

By reducing your meat consumption, you essentially take your foot off the gas pedal by inhibiting mTOR. This allows your body to relax and repair more often. Consequently, you'll get more mileage out of those old bones when you inhibit mTOR. That is why mTOR inhibition is associated with a longer lifespan.[115] [116]

So, you can eat meat, but probably not every day.

Things to consider regarding egg consumption:

Eating eggs will not raise your blood cholesterol. If the eggs come from healthy chickens, and if you are eating a well-rounded diet, you don't need to worry about an egg's cholesterol content. This is because dietary cholesterol does not directly raise the levels in your blood. Also, your body makes far more cholesterol than you could ever eat. We still don't know the whole story about cholesterol, but you can rest assured that egg consumption is not the problem.[117]

Still, according to the Blue Zones food guidelines (based on the longest-lived people in the world), the optimal egg intake is no more than three eggs per week.[118]

Also, various studies link egg consumption with diseases like prostate cancer and cardiovascular disease. We often blame choline for this association. If you are suffering from a similar condition, talk to your doctor. If you are eating an overall healthy diet, I wouldn't be scared about these potential side effects.

Things to consider regarding milk consumption:

Even if you are not lactose intolerant, you may notice that you feel bloated, gassy, or congested after consuming milk products. These symptoms are signs of inflammation, triggered by the casein-A1 proteins found in cow's milk. Essentially, excess casein-A1 protein means excess inflammation. Casein-A1 is to blame in most people, not lactose. Some scientists say that only a few people are lactose intolerant, but 75% of the world is dairy intolerant[119], probably due to the inflammatory effect of Casein-A1.

Also, consider what you are eating when you eat dairy. Cows make milk to feed their calves, which will grow to be over 300 pounds. Milk may be suitable for fast-growing babies, but do you need it as an adult? Even though milk has benefits, you can get the same benefits from many other food products. By cutting back on dairy, you won't be missing out on much.

However, if you can't cut back on dairy, look for casein-A2 milk products instead. Casein-A2 is not as inflammatory as casein-A1. These milk products come from animals such as goats, sheep, and water buffalo. Also, some imported cheeses from France or Italy contain casein-A2.

Habit Hacks:

- Create a habit contract by making the costs of the bad habit more public, painful, or visceral. For instance, every time you are about to buy an animal product, picture the slaughter of that animal. This may sound terrible, but the harsh reality is that eating another animal requires killing it, too; don't lose sight of that. You don't need to become vegan; just be intentional with your decisions. You are an animal eating another animal, and this is the natural way of life, but you should still respect the tremendous sacrifice that was made for your sustenance. Consequently, you'll still eat meat, but probably far less of it. Luckily, this pays dividends for your health and your wallet.

- Join a group that values regenerative agriculture, humane animal practices, and wild game. Usually, these groups consist of farmers, hunters, environmental groups, or various diet tribes (pescatarian, paleo, keto, etc.). Hanging out with people whose values align with your habits will help those habits stick a bit better.

- Cook in batches. I like to boil a dozen eggs, peel them immediately, and put them back in the carton. Then, when I'm in a rush, I can just grab a couple from the fridge for a hearty and nutritious midday snack. Putting baking soda in your fridge will help with the smell.

Tips & Tricks:

- If you don't know whether an animal product came from a well-raised, healthy animal, opt for the vegetarian or plant-based option instead. At most, choose an egg option. Unless you are splurging, it's just not worth it if the animal isn't healthy.

- To help you determine if an animal was raised humanely, look for the labels "**animal welfare approved**," "**American grass-fed association**," or "**organic**." You can also check out these resources: localharvest.org; eatwild.com; firsthandfoods.org; americangrassfed.org; thrivemarket.com

- Not all plant-based products are good for you or the environment. The soy farms that supply products for soy-based meat alternatives are often energy-intensive and unsustainable. Meanwhile, meat products from regenerative farms have a much smaller environmental impact. Therefore, meat isn't the bad guy, but the way we have been producing meat has gotten a bit out of control.

- Reheat meats and starchy foods in an oven or stovetop. Heating food in a microwave increases the production of advanced glycation end products (AGEs).[120] AGEs cause internal crusting or charring in your body. Aptly named, AGEs are associated with early aging.

WILD-CAUGHT SEAFOOD

Best of the best: small fish (anchovies, sardines, herring), salmon, mackerel, other seafood (clams, oysters, mollusks, mussels)

SELF-REGULATION	STRUCTURE & MOBILITY	MICROBIOME	IMMUNE BALANCE	ANGIOGENIC BALANCE	DNA REPAIR & ANTIOXIDANTS	REGENERATION & AUTOPHAGY	DETOX & EXCRETION	STRESS MGMT.
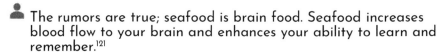								
✔	✔	✔	✔	✔	✔	✔	✔	✔

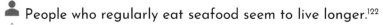 = the food is beneficial to the associated healing system

The rumors are true; seafood is brain food. Seafood increases blood flow to your brain and enhances your ability to learn and remember.[121]

People who regularly eat seafood seem to live longer.[122]

When you eat small fish like sardines, you eat their tiny bones, too. This gives you a ton of calcium and collagen for building strong bones and sturdy tissues.

Healthy fats in fish help support your microbiome.[123]

Pacific oysters increase your number of natural killer cells and T-cells to help you fight infections.[124] Oysters also help you make glutathione, your most potent antioxidant.[125]

Fish oil decreases inflammation.[126]

Seafood is antiangiogenic due to EPA/DHA fatty acids.[127]

Seafood helps improve your ability to protect and repair your DNA (e.g., oysters, sea cucumbers, clams, cockles, tuna, and yellowtail).[128]

Fish oil activates and improves the circulation of stem cells used for muscle regeneration and blood vessel regeneration.[129]

Many seafood dishes are rich in sulfur and B12, which help you sulfate and methylate toxins during detoxification.

Fish oil helps you deal with stress. Specifically, EPA and DHA lower norepinephrine levels and reduce cortisol spikes.[130]

Habit Hacks:

- Choose a fish day. Eating fish at least one day per week can boost your longevity. So, designate a day of the week when you will cook fish. May I suggest Friday?
- Some people don't like the taste of seafood. If so, just eat one bite per day. Keep your seafood meal in a Tupperware and put one bite on your plate at dinner time. This will help develop your taste buds to tolerate the "fishiness." Also, by trying many different types of seafood, you may find a dish that you enjoy. Never miss twice, though. If you forget your bite one day, make sure you get back on track tomorrow. It's just one bite; you can do it.

Tips & Tricks:

- Smaller fish are best due to their low mercury content and high nutritional density. Mercury accumulates as you go higher up in the fish food chain. Big fish like tuna have a high risk of mercury toxicity. Use the NRDC Smart Seafood Buying Guide to help you choose healthy fish with few toxins or pollutants.
- Look for the labels "**Aquaculture Stewardship Council**" or "**Antibiotic-free**" when buying fish. These labels ensure that proper fishery practices were met.
- If you are worried about over-fishing, check out the following TED talk: "The four fish we are over-eating and what to eat instead."
- Flash-frozen fish may preserve nutrients better than fresh fish because they freeze the fish immediately after catching it.
- Most people associate omega-3 fatty acids with fish, but fish get those fats from the green plants they eat (e.g., seaweed and algae). Seaweed and algae are so good for you that they deserve their own category. But since they are a little tough to stomach, consider supplementing with powdered algae or algae flakes. Green, brown, or red seaweed is the best, preferably from Canada or Maine.

NUTS & SEEDS

Best of the best: raw nuts (pistachio, macadamia, almond, hazelnut)

Self-Regulation	Structure & Mobility	Microbiome	Immune Balance	Angiogenic Balance	DNA Repair & Antioxidants	Regeneration & Autophagy	Detox & Excretion	Stress Mgmt.
✔		✔	✔	✔	✔	✔	✔	

✔ = the food is beneficial to the associated healing system

👤 Nuts and seeds are packed with essential nutrients to bring life into this world. If they can do that for a plant, then they're probably pretty dang good for you.

👤 Sesame, sunflower, and poppy seeds contain many omega-6 fatty acids. Omega 6's can be inflammatory, but they are also necessary for cellular health; they create support for cell walls, and they help with blood clotting.

👤 Pumpkin, chia, hemp, and flax seeds contain omega-3 fats to help with brain and eye health.[131]

👤 Nuts and seeds may improve cardiovascular function by regulating your blood pressure and lowering blood lipid levels.[132]

👤 Pistachios, cashews, almonds, macadamia nuts, and hazelnuts contain omega-9 fats. These fats are valuable for your brain and nervous system.[133]

🐞 Nuts and seeds feed your gut microbiome, primarily due to their insane fiber content.[134]

✳ One handful of tree nuts per day boosts your immune system and helps control inflammation.[135]
Examples of tree nuts: walnuts, pecans, almonds, cashews, pistachios, pine nuts, and macadamia

◈ Flaxseed, sunflower, sesame[136], pumpkin, and chia seeds contain lignans that stimulate angiogenesis and improve healing.[137]

◈ Tree nuts contain potent antiangiogenic omega-3 PUFA's.[138]

For every 10g of nuts or seeds that you eat, you could lengthen your telomeres by 8.5 base pairs.[139] Normally, your telomeres shorten by 15.4 base pairs per year. So, a handful of nuts per day slowed cell aging by 1.5 years.

Peanuts and pistachios (via resveratrol) activate cardiac stem cells that usually lie dormant in the heart.[140] It is nearly impossible to eat enough resveratrol to have these effects, though, so you may need to supplement it.

Chestnuts and walnuts act as stem cell activators (via ellagic acid).[141]

Nuts and seeds have plenty of fiber, which means better bowel movements and better excretion capabilities.

Cashews and peanuts have lots of magnesium, thereby helping you detoxify more effectively.

Brazil nuts, peanuts, and almonds promote the sulfation of toxins during phase II of liver detoxification.

Habit Hacks:

- Eat one handful of nuts per day. Form this habit by writing down a specific time and place where this behavior will occur. For example, when you make coffee in the morning, grab one handful of nuts from the cupboard. You are not committing to eating the nuts; you are just grabbing a handful from the cupboard. It's a gateway habit, a tiny habit that helps start the ritual. The key is never to break the streak. Even if you only end up eating one nut, you kept the habit alive.

Tips & Tricks:

- If raw nuts are hard to come by, roasted or baked nuts are fine. Just watch out for sugars and other added ingredients. There is no reason why a nut should have more than five ingredients. Interestingly, roasted peanuts are better than raw peanuts because roasting brings out more resveratrol.
- Grains, legumes, nuts, and seeds contain phytates, which limit your ability to absorb certain nutrients (aka anti-nutrients). But, if you soak them in water for at least 24 hours before consuming them, you can eliminate their anti-nutrient effect.

LEGUMES

Best of the best: black beans, lentils, soy

Self-Regulation	Structure & Mobility	Microbiome	Immune Balance	Angiogenic Balance	DNA Repair & Antioxidants	Regeneration & Autophagy	Detox & Excretion	Stress Mgmt.
✓		✓	✓	✓	✓	✓	✓	

✓ = the food is beneficial to the associated healing system

- Almost all the longest-living cultures in the world eat beans as a staple in their diet. On average, they consume at least half a cup of beans per day.

- Soy is one of the only plant products that contain a full set of essential amino acids. Soy is the powerhouse of plant foods.

- Beans & legumes are highly prebiotic (via fiber).[142]

- Beans help thicken the layer of mucus coating your intestines, which protects and strengthens your gut lining.[143]

- There is some evidence that legumes have anti-inflammatory effects (via lectins and peptides).[144] However, soy is pro-inflammatory, so don't get too crazy with the soy burgers.

- Legumes are antiangiogenic (through isoflavones like genistein, daidzein, equol, and glyceollin).[145] [146]

- Soy epigenetically activates tumor suppressor genes, such as the BRCA gene mutation, to help fight breast cancer.[147] [148]

- Soy kills stem cells associated with prostate cancer.[149]

- The fiber in legumes improves bowel function for better toxin excretion.

- Beans contain many helpful nutrients to support liver detoxification, including quercetin, D-glucaric-acid, magnesium, sulfur, and folate.

- Lentils are rich in cysteine, which means increased production of your antioxidant powerhouse, glutathione.

Habit Hacks:

- Try eating one handful of beans per day. Try this habit hack: "every time I cook dinner for my family, I will put a handful of cooked beans on each plate."
- Cook a big batch of beans that you can use throughout the week. Heck, you could probably cook a batch for the whole month.
- Make beans visible. Don't put beans on the top shelf or in the back of the cupboard, away from view. Bring them to the front and center, along with your nuts and seeds. Let their presence be a constant reminder to eat one handful per day.

Tips & Tricks:

- The biological value of legumes is not as high as animal protein (soy = 74, other beans = <50), which means you won't absorb as much protein.[150] However, when you eat a combination of protein-rich plants, the biological value increases. For example, eating beans and rice will increase the BV significantly.[151]
- I don't recommend eating fake meat (like processed soy burgers or tofu hot dogs). These foods are Frankenfoods like any other processed junk. If you want a meat alternative, make it yourself. I like making black bean burgers by mashing black beans, mixing them with oats, and adding an egg or two.
- Grains, legumes, nuts, and seeds contain phytates, which limit your ability to absorb nutrients (aka antinutrients). But, if you soak the legumes in water for at least 24 hours, you can eliminate the anti-nutrient effect.[152] Although, if you pressure-cook your beans, you won't need to soak them ahead of time.
- Canned beans are quick to cook and are almost just as good as dry beans. Make sure they only contain a few ingredients, though, including beans, water, spices, and maybe a little salt. Avoid the canned beans that have added fat or sugar.

Side Note: Soy and Cancer

Soy does not cause breast cancer. People were concerned about soy because it chemically looks like estrogen. But we have recently discovered that soy does not have the same cancerous properties as other types of estrogens. Actually, soy is an antiestrogen that protects you against cancers that are fueled by excess estrogen.[153]

The best forms of soy are edamame, soy nuts, tempeh, miso, natto, soymilk, soy sauce, and tofu.

FUNGUS

Best of the best: porcini mushroom, white button mushroom

SELF-REGULATION	STRUCTURE & MOBILITY	MICROBIOME	IMMUNE BALANCE	ANGIOGENIC BALANCE	DNA PROTECTION &	REGENERATION & AUTOPHAGY	DETOX & EXCRETION	STRESS MGMT.
✔	✔	✔	✔		✔	✔	✔	

✔ = the food is beneficial to the associated healing system

👤 Vitamin D is essential for cellular function, calcium absorption, and sleep quality. Mushrooms are one of the few sources of ingestible vitamin D.[154]

👤 Mushrooms may be able to improve the function of your muscles and make you better at metabolizing energy.[155]

🐛 In all their fibrous glory, mushrooms are fuel for your microbiome. On top of that, mushrooms are typically grown in bacteria-rich soil, giving them probiotic qualities, too.[156] [157]

✳ White button and shiitake mushrooms contain immune-stimulating dietary fiber, which activates antibody secretion in your saliva.[158] [159] [160] [161]

✳ Truffles contain pheromones which boost immunity and act as a neurotransmitter to stimulate euphoria.[162] [163] [164]

🧬 Mushrooms protect your DNA.[165] Enough said.

🔄 The high concentration of polyamines in mushrooms may promote longevity.

☢ Mushrooms like Porcinis and white button mushrooms contain the most potent antioxidant, glutathione.

Tips & Tricks:

- Cook your mushrooms. Mushrooms have tough cell walls, making them difficult to digest. Cooking helps to break down those cell walls so you can absorb more nutrients. However, cooking causes some nutrient loss. The best way to preserve nutrients is to cook your mushrooms by microwave or grill.

- If you're interested, there is a world of information about medicinal and psychoactive mushrooms. Even if you don't care to consume them, I recommend learning more about mushrooms, lichen, and other fungi. You'll be stunned by the sophisticated and elaborate characteristics that these unique organisms exhibit. For instance, the "honey fungus" in Oregon is the largest organism in the world, covering 3.4 miles. Also, there are more than 75 species of mushrooms that glow in the dark.

Fermented Foods

Best of the best: sauerkraut, kimchi, tempeh (soy), miso, natto, yogurt, kefir, kombucha, pickled veggies, vinegar

Self-Regulation	Structure & Mobility	Microbiome	Immune Balance	Angiogenic Balance	DNA Repair & Antioxidants	Regeneration & Autophagy	Detox & Excretion	Stress Mgmt.
✓		✓	✓	✓	✓	✓	✓	✓

✓ = the food is beneficial to the associated healing system

👤 *Lactobacillus reuteri* is a common bacterial species found in fermented foods. This bacterium prevents the accumulation of abdominal fat, strengthens your hair, and improves your skin tone.[166]

👤 Kimchi helps improve glucose tolerance and digestion while optimizing your cholesterol, blood pressure, and body fat (via propionic acid and succinic acid).[167]

🦠 Fermented vegetables repopulate your gut (probiotic) and give your microbiome fibrous fuel to keep them healthy and functioning ideally (prebiotic). Some examples of fermented vegetables include sauerkraut, kimchi, pao cai, miso, and tempeh.

🦠 Research shows that natural foods influence microbial health more than probiotic supplements.[168] This is most likely because natural food offers a more diverse group of bacteria, some that we probably haven't discovered yet.

✳️ Some bacteria activate immune cells, while others down-regulate your immune system to prevent allergic reactions. Fermented foods help balance your microbiome and thus balance your immunity.

◈ Kimchi contains vitamin K2, which is antiangiogenic.

◈ *Lactobacillus reuteri* in fermented foods can help you heal faster by speeding up angiogenesis.[169]

Since your microbiome is intimately related to other self-healing processes, improvements in your gut flora (by eating fermented foods) lead to improved DNA repair, stem cell function, and immune function.

Lactobacillus plantarum in sauerkraut & pao cai produce isothiocyanates that kill cancerous stem cells and trigger an anti-inflammatory response in your intestinal stem cells.[170]

The bacteria in fermented vegetables (*Lactobacillus reuteri*) stimulate oxytocin production to improve social bonding. Social bonding significantly decreases your stress response and improves mental health.[171]

Tips & Tricks:

- Make your own kombucha! It is super easy to make, and you can flavor it with fresh foods like ginger and many fruits. The most challenging part is finding a SCOBY, which is the starter culture of bacteria. It looks like a soggy pancake. Usually, you can buy a SCOBY online or borrow a layer from a friend.

OIL

Best of the best: extra virgin olive oil (EVOO), coconut, flaxseed

SELF-REGULATION	STRUCTURE & MOBILITY	MICROBIOME	IMMUNE BALANCE	ANGIOGENIC BALANCE	DNA REPAIR & ANTIOXIDANTS	REGENERATION & AUTOPHAGY	DETOX & EXCRETION	STRESS MGMT.
✔	✔	✔	✔	✔		✔	✔	

✔ = the food is beneficial to the associated healing system

Flaxseed is high in plant-based omega-3 fatty acids (such as ALA), which invigorate your gut lining.[172][173] Flaxseed also contains lignans and vitamins that are essential for cell function.

Coconut oil contains saturated fats, which are an essential component in your cell membranes. We used to think saturated fat was bad for cardiovascular health. However, it turns out that coconut oil raises our cardio-protective HDL cholesterol levels.[174] In the 'Foods to Limit' section, you'll see that the real problem with saturated fat is when we combine it with sugars and carbohydrates.

Extra virgin olive oil (EVOO) may help to prevent bone loss.[175]

Omega-3 fats from flaxseed and olive oil can prevent muscle loss as you age.[176]

Flaxseed oil contains prebiotic fiber, and the omega-3 fats are bug food, too.[177]

EVOO improves your microbiome diversity.[178]

EVOO increases T cell activation and has potent anti-inflammatory effects (via oleocanthal).[179] The polyphenols in olive oil are also anti-cancerous.[180]

Omega-3's in flaxseed oil help down-regulate inflammation and balance out the pro-inflammatory effect of some omega-6 fats.[181]

Coconut oil has anti-infective properties.[182] Mostly, this effect comes from using coconut oil as an emollient to rub on your skin. I imagine a similar effect occurs by ingesting coconut oil, though.

Olive oil has bioactive polyphenols that are antiangiogenic.[183]

Flaxseed oil's high omega-3 concentration helps support cardiovascular health by making blood vessels more flexible and reducing atherosclerotic plaque buildup.[184]

EVOO helps kickstart autophagy so you can recycle old cells and usher in new and healthy cells[185]

EVOO and coconut oil protect your brain from amyloid toxicity (and, consequently, Alzheimer's disease).[186 187]

EVOO keeps your detox system running smoothly by protecting your liver in several ways.[188]

Habit Hacks:

- Coconut oil, EVOO, and butter from a healthy animal. With these three items, you can cook almost any meal you want. Get rid of everything else, so you aren't tempted to use it. Then, use your olive and coconut oil like crazy. Put it on salads, vegetables, potatoes, meat; you name it. These fats will give your food an extra dose of health as well as a flavor explosion!

Tips & Tricks:

- When choosing olive oil, do the 3-cough test. The more "peppery" tasting the oil, the higher the oil quality. If you cough three times after swallowing a spoonful, you've got yourself a top-notch olive oil.

- Each time you heat oil, the oil breaks down into oxidizing agents, which can damage your DNA. If your oil starts smoking, you have overheated it. Start over. And depending on the temperature of your cooking surface, you should use a different type of oil. Use the chart below as a guide. The best oils for your health are bolded.

High Heat (>450)	Medium heat (400-450)	Low heat (<400)
Red palm (unrefined)	**Coconut (unrefined)**	**Butter** (from a healthy animal)
Almond/peanut (refined)	**EVOO**	**Lard** (from a healthy animal)
Avocado (refined)	Canola/soybean (refined)	Sesame/Sunflower (unrefined)
Grapeseed (refined)		

CERTAIN GRAINS (BUT NOT MUCH)

Best of the best: quinoa, oatmeal, sourdough, pumpernickel, rice bran

SELF-REGULATION	STRUCTURE & MOBILITY	MICROBIOME	IMMUNE BALANCE	ANGIOGENIC BALANCE	DNA REPAIR & ANTIOXIDANTS	REGENERATION & AUTOPHAGY	DETOX & EXCRETION	STRESS MGMT.
✔		✔	✔	✔	✔	✔		✔

✔ = the food is beneficial to the associated healing system

Sourdough's acidic nature degrades the phytates that are in most bread. Phytates reduce the absorption of healthy vitamins and minerals, but since sourdough has low phytate levels, you absorb more nutrients. Consequently, your cells get more fuel than they would from conventional bread.[189]

Sourdough and pumpernickel have *Lactobacillus reuteri* bacteria in the starter batch, which helps reduce weight gain and speeds up wound healing.[190] *Lactobacillus* also digest the wheat proteins within a slice of sourdough bread, so it may contain less gluten than the products labeled "gluten-free." If you are gluten-intolerant, you may be able to handle sourdough, rye, or pumpernickel bread.[191]

Lactobacillus in sourdough helps improve immune function.[192]

Rice bran (aka the leftover stuff when converting brown rice to white rice) helps repair damaged blood vessels (via bio-actives). One concern for rice bran is that it contains a small amount of arsenic.

During fermentation, the bacteria in sourdough bread release antioxidants, which protect your DNA from damage.[193] Rye and Pumpernickel bread also contain antioxidants.[194]

Rice bran has dietary fiber and bio-actives, which protect and increase the survival of endothelial stem cells.[195]

The bacteria in Sourdough stimulate oxytocin, thereby improving social bonding and mental health while decreasing stress.[196]

Habit Hacks:

- Grains are not necessary for your health, and some doctors suggest that the food pyramid/MyPlate should not include the 'grains' category at all.[197] Therefore, you don't need to make a habit out of eating grains. In fact, you may want to discontinue your bread and pasta-eating habit altogether. To avoid the habit of eating too much bread and grain, try these strategies:
  - o Remove the cues from your environment. Does seeing deli meat in the fridge trigger your desire to make a sandwich? Then don't keep bread and deli meat in the house. Instead, change your idea of what a sandwich looks like. Eat lettuce wraps for lunch or use slices of meat in place of bread.
  - o Reframe your mindset. Instead of thinking about the sacrifices, highlight the benefits of avoiding grains and bread. For example, abstaining from unhealthy grains keeps you more energized throughout the day, you aren't hungry as much, and you stay more focused and productive.
  - o Every time you abstain from eating grains, reward yourself. Consider setting up a sandwich savings account. Every time you resist a deli sandwich, transfer the cost of that sandwich from your checking to a savings account. After a while, you can buy yourself a reward from your savings.

Tips & Tricks

- No matter what kind of bread you are eating, the homemade version is almost always better than store-bought products. Learn to make bread yourself, and you can feel good about eating it rather than worrying about all the carbs and unhealthy stuff. Plus, the acting of kneading the dough is excellent exercise.
- Gluten-free does not mean healthy. Dried or pulverized starches within gluten-free foods will raise your blood sugar just as much as other flours. So, don't just replace wheat with gluten-free replicas. Junk is still junk, even if it doesn't have gluten in it.
  Examples of gluten-free flours: corn starch, rice starch, potato starch, tapioca starch, amaranth, arrowroot, buckwheat, bean flour, hominy grits, and polenta.

EATING STRATEGIES

Remember, this is not a diet book. However, a few eating strategies are gaining scientific clout and popularity, so I'd like to address their benefits. It is important to note that, for a healthy population, these are not long-term diets. These are short-term diets intended to stimulate healing in your body.

Also, note that the way you consume food is almost as important as *what* you consume. One of the best eating strategies is to prepare a meal with a group of people (e.g., your family) and eat it together. Dan Buettner's study of the people who live the longest showed that nearly every long-lived culture would cook food for friends and family and spend time enjoying the meal with them.[198] Even though these cultures had vastly different diets, the way they ate was probably the most critical factor for their longevity.

So, how are you consuming *your* food? Are you cooking and eating with loved ones, or are you cramming down a fast-food meal so you can get going with the rest of your day?

Best of the best: fasting-mimicking diet, time-restricted feeding, ketosis (for short periods)

	Self-Regulation	Structure & Mobility	Microbiome	Immune Balance	Angiogenic Balance	DNA Repair & Antioxidants	Regeneration & Autophagy	Detox & Excretion	Stress Mgmt.
Fasting Mimicking	✓	✓	✓	✓	✓	✓	✓	✓	
Time-Restricted Feeding	✓	✓	✓	✓	✓	✓	✓	✓	
Ketosis Diet	✓	✓	✓	✓	✓	✓	✓	✓	

✓ = the food is beneficial to the associated healing system

Calorie Restriction & Fasting

There are many ways to restrict calories, but they all have the same fundamental goal. Calorie restriction creates controlled stress on your body, called hormesis. Your body thinks it needs to prepare for an upcoming fast, so it gets rid of the old and worn-out cells and keeps the strong cells that can handle an upcoming challenge.

The most popular calorie restriction strategies include the fasting-mimicking diet (by Valter Longo) and intermittent fasting (more accurately described as time-restricted feeding).

The official fasting-mimicking diet entails eating 900 calories (of a mostly vegan diet) each day for five days. According to Dr. Longo, this five day fast should occur roughly once per month.[199]

Comparatively, the typical time-restricted feeding diet includes eating for 12 hours in the day and not eating for the remaining 12 hours. An overly simplified explanation is to eat when it's light outside and don't eat after 7 pm.

The key to a good fast is to make sure you end your fast with very high quality, healthy food. If not, you risk undoing all the progress you made during the fast. Eating sugar immediately after ending your fast is one of the worst things you can do.

Side Note: My fasting strategy

I'll be honest; I have never actually done the fasting-mimicking diet. However, I write about it because it has the most research to substantiate its effects. For my fasting strategy, I only drink water (zero calories) for 24-72 hrs. I do this 3-4 times per year as a biological reset.

Below are some examples of the benefits gained from controlled caloric restriction or fasting. For more information on these fasting strategies, check out the links in the 'Resources' section of the appendix.

Calorie restriction remains the most robust method for extending lifespan and healthspan in every biological model.[200] If you want to live longer and healthier, fasting is the single greatest tool in your toolkit.

During a prolonged fast, your organs literally shrink in size. When you re-feed (with high-quality food), the organs grow back to their standard size with a new batch of young and vibrant cells.[201]

The fasting-mimicking diet leads to fat loss and muscle loss. However, when you re-feed (with high-quality food), your body prioritizes muscle mass while avoiding fat production.[202]

Fasting decreases the growth and reproduction of bacterial populations. After all, you are starving your bacteria, too. Therefore, the strongest bacteria will survive the starvation, and your entire microbiome will be more resilient afterward.

Fasting strengthens the protective mucosal lining of your gut, therefore making it less likely for foreign objects to get into your body and cause inflammation.[203] [204]

Some animal studies show that calorie restriction can improve wound repair via angiogenic stimulation.[205]

When you eat, your body focuses on digestion. When you don't eat, your body can devote its free time to repairing the parts of a cell, such as fixing broken strands of DNA.

20-40% reduction in calories can regenerate your gut by activating stem cells in the crypts of your intestines.[206]

Fasting for 2-4 days forces the body to go into autophagy/recycling mode. When you reintroduce good food, hematopoietic stem cells are activated to refresh your immune cell populations.[207] [208] [209]

When you fast, your body isn't using energy to digest food (which is a costly process). Instead, your body uses the energy to clean up your shop and repair damaged areas. For instance, while you're sleeping (and not eating, of course), your body power washes your brain and cleans out the toxins that build up throughout the day.

Ketogenic diet

Ketosis is a state in which your body is using ketones to make energy. Ketones are a product of fat breakdown, and they act as an alternative fuel for your cells. When your cells don't have access to glucose, they look for ketones to get their energy.

Many people try to achieve ketosis by dramatically reducing their carbohydrate intake. Carbs turn into glucose. So, restricting carbohydrates will decrease cellular glucose levels. Then, without glucose around, your cells are more likely to use ketones for energy.

Ketones are a fabulous energy source because they are highly efficient, they have unique effects on the brain, and they starve cancer cells (cancer loves glucose, but it can't use ketones).

However, you don't want to be in ketosis all the time. You want to be more like a hybrid car, switching between fuel sources as needed. Sometimes you'll want to burn ketones, but glucose should be your primary fuel. This ability to change between fuel sources is called metabolic flexibility, and it helps your cells maintain optimal function. If your body relies on only one energy source, you will be less adaptable to physical stressors. Consequently, those stressors will cause more damaging effects over time. But when your cells are metabolically flexible, they can be more resilient and adaptable to your ever-changing internal environment.

You probably don't need to worry about ketosis at this stage in your health journey. But feel free to review the benefits of ketosis below. Once you've mastered the basics of Lifelong Youth, then you can start working on this diet strategy.

- Your brain cells love using ketones as alternative energy. The ketogenic diet has shown exceptional efficacy in treating epilepsy.[210] Also, ketones may be neuroprotective against Alzheimer's.[211]

- The ketogenic diet is often used for weight loss because it is very safe and highly effective.[212]

- The ketogenic diet has shown to be effective at treating epilepsy through its interaction with the gut microbiota, too.[213] For non-epileptic people, these microbiome changes may optimize your brain health and the communication between your gut and brain.

- The ketones produced through ketosis have anti-inflammatory effects,[214] which partially explains why a ketogenic diet improves Alzheimer's disease.[215]

- A ketogenic diet has anti-cancer properties by inhibiting angiogenesis and tumor cell growth.[216]

- Ketones are anti-oxidative, which helps protect your DNA.[217]

- Ketone helps fine-tune your intestinal stem cells by training them to be more adaptable in different environments (aka maintain homeostasis).[218]

Habit Hacks:

- Get a fasting buddy. It's easier to fast with a friend.
- Before starting your fast, do something you enjoy. Maybe you go to a nice restaurant. Or maybe you invite your friends over to serve them your first ketosis meal. Choose an activity that is meaningful to you or one that might give you a boost of motivation.

Tips & Tricks:

- While fasting, drink a lot of water. I mean it, over a gallon per day.
- Hara hachi bu - Eat until you are 80% full. You don't need to stuff yourself at every meal. Eat until you're satisfied, not bloated.
- Get smaller plates to limit your portion size. Research shows that people will eat 30% more when given bigger portions of food.[219]
- When you eat alone, just eat. Don't watch shows or scroll through your phone; this leads to mindless over-eating.
- Make cooking an exercise. Blend, whisk, and open cans by hand; don't use those electric imposters. Then, share your meals with friends and family. Doing things by hand burns calories, and eating together increases your longevity.

SUPPLEMENTS

Sometimes, your diet needs a little boost. Even if you're eating a lot of nutritionally dense food, you won't always get everything you need to support optimal cell function. So, in order to optimize, supplements can be useful.

Unfortunately, supplements are often misused. Instead of "supplementing" an already healthy diet, people eat bad food all day and think a supplement will make up for it. But you cannot use supplements to avoid eating well.

The only way to achieve Lifelong Youth is if you eat whole food. Whole foods have so much more nutrient complexity than supplements. They contain an array of substances that interact with your cells in unique ways, while supplements are just isolated nutrients. Whole Foods play Beethoven's fifth symphony in your body. Supplements play chopsticks.

So, start with whole foods, then use supplements to take your health to the next level.

On the following pages, you'll find some supplement suggestions that might help you optimize your health. These suggestions are based on common nutrient deficiencies that American's experience. However, you are a unique individual. Before taking any of these supplements, talk to your doctor or health professional. Also, get your blood tested for nutrient deficiencies. If you have optimal nutrient levels, taking supplements could be toxic.

Side Note: The Multivitamin

Daily multivitamins make for expensive pee.

If you've ever taken a multivitamin, you may have noticed that your pee turns a bright yellow or slightly greenish color. This is because most of the nutrients in multivitamins are water-soluble, so they pass through your body quickly. Many nutrients don't get absorbed, and the unabsorbed nutrients get peed out.

It is not harmful to pee out the nutrients, but you paid good money for that supplement, so you probably don't want your money to go down the toilet. However, if you value the proverbial "insurance policy" that a multivitamin provides, then go for it. A multivitamin may be a simple way to fulfill your nutrient needs.

Supplement	Notes
B complex	A healthy diet will give you plenty of B-vitamins. But it may behoove you to take a supplement because B-vitamins are crucial for energy metabolism, nervous system function, protein synthesis, DNA synthesis, collagen production, and many more cellular functions.
	If you are worried about having the MTHFR gene, consider the methylated forms of vitamins B12 and B9. The MTHFR genetic mutation impacts how well you detoxify, and it may limit the effectiveness of some B-vitamins. Taking methyl-B12/cobalamin and methyl-B9/folate means the vitamins are already methylated, and they will be more effective in your body. Since about 25% of the population carries the MTHFR gene, you might want to take methylated B-vitamins regardless of whether you know you are a carrier or not.
Vitamin C	Vit C is a powerhouse vitamin that we recognize as an immune booster. But it also plays a role in building collagen, which means strong tendons, ligaments, and youthful skin.
	This supplement is unique because the synthetic form is the same as the natural form. Therefore, it is absorbed the same way and has the same function in the body.
	However, one cup of broccoli has more Vit C than your typical supplement, so if you are already eating foods high in Vit C, you don't need to supplement it. To avoid diarrhea, keep your vitamin C intake below 2,000mg/day.
Vitamin D	For people living in Northern climates, supplementing with vitamin D may be necessary. But, if you spend 15 minutes in the sun, you have produced enough vitamin D for the day, and you do not need a supplement. Sunscreen, though, blocks vitamin D absorption.
	Every cell in your body has a receptor for vitamin D, which speaks to this vitamin's importance.

Supplement	Notes
Vitamin E	This vitamin helps repair your connective tissues and enhances oxygen utilization by the body. So, it may be useful to take vitamin E during periods of intense exercise or sport.
Vitamin K2	K2 is an excellent supplement to take in combination with vitamin D.
	When you feel dental plaque buildup behind your teeth (called dental calculus), it is a sign that you don't have enough vitamin K2. It also may be an indicator of calcium imbalance.
	When you eat leafy greens and organ meat, your gut bacteria make a version of vitamin K called NK7.
Fish oil or Omega-3 oil	Fish oil is another term for concentrated EPA & DHA fatty acids. If you can't stand seafood, are a vegetarian, or if you're worried about mercury toxicity in fish, this is a valid option. Just know that eating real seafood is far more effective than the supplement.
	Cod Liver Oil is an old version of fish oil, and it has higher levels of vitamins D and A. It tastes and smells like fish, but if you can swallow it, it may be an even healthier option.
	Some high-quality fish oil options are <u>Green Pasture's</u> fermented fish liver oil or highly concentrated, molecularly distilled fish oil (<u>Nordic Naturals</u> or <u>Solgar</u> brand)
CoQ10 N-acetylcysteine L-Carnitine	These nutrients help enhance mitochondrial function.
Choline	Vegans and vegetarians are often deficient in choline. Choline also helps with memory and learning.
Pre & Probiotics	These may be important to take after you've been on a round of antibiotics.

Supplement	Notes
Magnesium	People are commonly deficient in this useful mineral, but it is found naturally in beans, greens, nuts, and seeds. I like taking a combination of Calcium, Magnesium, and Potassium
Calcium	Calcium helps build bone, but you won't absorb much calcium if you are not exercising regularly. I recommend calcium citrate because you can take it with or without food.
Selenium	Selenium acts as an indirect antioxidant by helping to produce your most potent antioxidant, glutathione. You could also take liposomal glutathione for direct access to this supercharged antioxidant.
Resveratrol	Resveratrol is a mitochondria booster found in wine and grapes. However, there isn't much resveratrol in grapes, so supplementation is necessary if you are interested in optimizing this polyphenol.
Lectin Shield	This substance helps you stop lectins from getting through your gut lining and causing inflammation.
Digestive enzymes	These proteins help support gut health by aiding digestion. These may be especially useful if you have a food intolerance to foods like wheat, dairy, soy, eggs, nuts, fish, hemp, & peas.
Rapamycin/Rapa-logs	In animal and human studies, rapamycin inhibited the mTOR gene and increased longevity as a result.[220] [221] These effects are similar to those seen after fasting and calorie restriction.

Foods to Limit

I know I said this book wasn't going to be about sacrifices, but I would be remiss if I didn't steer you away from the toxic foods in your world. I don't want you to feel like you are suffering, so I will not ask you to give up these foods entirely. However, you must know that your journey to Lifelong Youth will be significantly hindered if you continue to eat these foods in excess.

The toxic foods I'm talking about are corn, sugar, wheat flour, and "sweet" saturated fats. Or, I could just say processed junk. I won't even give these items the respect of calling them food because they are not. They are Frankenfoods, with no resemblance to plants or whole food. Unfortunately, this processed junk shows up in our grocery stores more than any other item, which is why we end up eating too much of it.

In all fairness, corn, sugar, wheat, and saturated fats are not the enemy. In their natural form and in natural amounts, these foods can be healthy additions to your life. But as the processed food industry brought these foods out of the farm and into the laboratory, they stripped away the nutritional qualities.

Although food processing may have started with good intentions, those intentions quickly turned diabolical. Despite all the research showing the dangers of these processed foods, the food industry kept making these toxic products because "it's what people are buying." Meanwhile, the big food companies were concocting recipes specifically engineered to make their foods more addictive and irresistible. They then hired the smartest business marketers in the world to prey on our society's innocent minds, getting our kids and less-educated citizens hooked on these new drugs.

As a result, the grocery stores started filling up with processed Frankenfoods. And junk food marketers disguised their garbage behind attractive labels and claims of good health. In no time at all, Americans became some of the fattest and unhealthiest in the world, even though we were exercising more than ever before.

Ultimately, the biggest reason Americans are so unhealthy today is that we keep over-eating the same four ingredients: corn, sugar, wheat, and sweet saturated fat. In the following pages, you'll see why these four foods can be so detrimental to your health.

CORN

Corn is everywhere. High fructose corn syrup, corn-fed beef, maltodextrin, corn starch, magazine covers, and even packing peanuts are just a few examples of hidden corn. In an average grocery store (with 45,000 food items), about 1/4 of the goods sold contain corn.

With all this corn around, it's no wonder why Americans eat a lot of it. The average American eats a ton of corn every year, mostly in the form of corn-fed meat and processed foods.

Corn is not all bad, though. It is a plant, after all, and it has some benefits when eaten in the whole form. But remember, the problem is dosage. Even medicine becomes poisonous when you take too much of it. And since corn is so ubiquitous in the American grocery store, we end up eating way too much of it. By limiting your corn consumption, you are still likely to find it hidden somewhere in your diet. But hopefully, you'll be eating it in much smaller quantities, so you won't experience as many damaging effects as described below.

SELF-REGULATION	STRUCTURE & MOBILITY	MICROBIOME	IMMUNE BALANCE	ANGIOGENIC BALANCE	DNA REPAIR & ANTIOXIDANTS	REGENERATION & AUTOPHAGY	DETOX & EXCRETION	STRESS MGMT.
	✗	✗	✗					

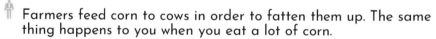 = the food is potentially harmful to the associated healing system

Farmers feed corn to cows in order to fatten them up. The same thing happens to you when you eat a lot of corn.

If you eat a lot of corn, your corn-hungry bacterial species will thrive while your other healthy species may suffer, thus creating an imbalanced microbiome.

Omega-6 fats help you heal by initiating inflammation. However, excess omega-6 intake causes excess inflammation, which leads to collateral damage to healthy cells.[222] You usually want a 1:1 balance between omega-6 and omega-3 fats, but corn products have a ratio of roughly 60:1.[223]

Artificial Sweeteners, Fructose, & High Sugar

Self-Regulation	Structure & Mobility	Microbiome	Immune Balance	Angiogenic Balance	DNA Repair & Antioxidants	Regeneration & Autophagy	Detox & Excretion	Stress Mgmt.
X	X	X	X		X	X	X	

✗ = the food is potentially harmful to the associated healing system

👤 Fructose from non-fruit sources may make your cells more insulin resistant.[224] This means more glucose will stay in your blood, which can cause damage to your kidneys, nerves, and eyes.

👤 Fructose is addictive.[225] It stimulates the same reward response in our brain as cocaine, meth, opiates, and other drugs.

🧍 Fructose delays the release of your satiety hormone, ghrelin.[226] [227] Consequently, you'll keep eating without feeling full. Then, fructose stimulates your production of fat, triglycerides, and LDL cholesterol. Basically, excess fructose intake is a recipe for obesity.

🧍 Fructose is toxic to the liver, just like alcohol. Consequently, fructose is a significant contributor to non-alcoholic fatty liver disease.[228]

🐞 Some bacterial species thrive off sugars, while others like different foods. By eating too many sugars and carbs, your sugar-loving bacteria will increase while the other populations will diminish, thus creating an imbalance in your microbiome.

🐞 Artificial sweeteners may negatively impact your good bacteria.[229] They also negatively affect your glucose tolerance[230] and contribute to weight gain. Ironically, sweeteners were designed to reduce these harmful effects. Oops.

✳ Excess sugar and carb intake trigger the production of advanced glycation end-products (AGEs). Aptly named, AGEs make you age faster and put you at risk for age-related chronic diseases. Like rust inside your body, AGEs stiffen joints (arthritis), accumulate in the eyes (cataracts), and cause havoc in the brain (dementia). Fructose is 7-10 times more likely to produce AGEs than glucose,[231] and other added sugars will increase your development of AGEs, too.[232]

✕ Sugary beverages can shorten your telomeres. People that drank 21 ounces of soda per day for one year had shorter lifespans by 4.6 years.[233]

↻ Foods that spike your blood sugar also impair stem cell activation, mobilization, and production (in endothelial, bone, and cardiac stem cells).[234] [235] [236]

☢ Fructose hijacks your liver. Every time you eat fructose, your liver focuses all its energy on detoxifying just the fructose. Meanwhile, the rest of the toxins in your body get backed up. So, if you're eating fructose all the time (eghm, high fructose corn syrup), the toxin traffic jam can cause inflammatory chaos.

WHEAT FLOUR

SELF-REGULATION	STRUCTURE & MOBILITY	MICROBIOME	IMMUNE BALANCE	ANGIOGENIC BALANCE	DNA REPAIR & ANTIOXIDANTS	REGENERATION & AUTOPHAGY	DETOX & EXCRETION	STRESS MGMT.
✗	✗	✗	✗					

✗ = the food is potentially harmful to the associated healing system

👤 Many people think that grains give you fiber, but we destroy the fiber when we pulverize grains into flour. In fact, without wheat, people tend to eat MORE fiber via fruits and veggies.

👤 Wheat contains a substance called wheat germ agglutinin (WGA). When WGA gets into your blood, it can trigger fat production. It also blocks glucose from getting into your nerve and muscle cells, causing sarcopenia (muscle wasting) and nerve dysfunction.

🧍 Flour is extremely easy to digest, but this means that the glucose within flour is absorbed very quickly. Consequently, when you eat flour, you get a massive spike in blood sugar. Your body doesn't like a lot of sugar in your blood, so it will try to shove all the extra glucose into fat cells. Typically, your body stores this excess sugar in the fat cells around your belly, thus covering your organs in fat, and reducing their function (aka visceral fat).

🐛 Wheat is a relatively recent addition to the human diet, so our microbiome may suffer if we eat too many grains and flours.

✹ Wheat ingestion is associated with the phenomenon called "leaky gut" (aka intestinal permeability). When you eat wheat, tiny bits of undigested food can sneak through your gut wall and enter your bloodstream. Your body thinks these undigested fragments are foreign invaders, so it launches an immune attack, causing unnecessary inflammation and damages your healthy cells.[237]

✹ Visceral fat (as discussed above) can act like a gland and produce hormones that trigger unnecessary inflammation.[238]

"Sweet" Saturated Fats

Saturated fats were once vilified because we thought they contributed to heart disease. But now we know that saturated fats are not as bad as we once thought.

Saturated fats have many beneficial effects. For example, breast milk is loaded with saturated fat because it is good for the brain and immune system development.[239]

However, there are still some saturated fats that we should limit. Dr. Mark Hyman calls them "sweet fats." Sweet fat means that a food contains high carbohydrates in addition to saturated fat. You could also call them "junk food" or "splurge foods" because sweet fats are mostly found in things like donuts, ice cream, French fries, and cookies.

Junk foods aren't the only source of sweet fats, though. A diet with lots of processed animal products, in addition to processed carbs, may create the same problems as junk food. This is because animal products are a major source of saturated fat, and processed carbs are a major sugar source. Hence, you'll have sugars and fats in the same meal, much like the junk food described above.

So, if you're going to eat a diet high in saturated fats, you shouldn't be eating processed carbs and sugar, too. Thankfully, there is a loophole. If the carbs and sugars in your diet come from vegetables and fruit, saturated fats are more helpful than harmful. Better yet, if you get your saturated fats from healthy, minimally processed animal products, you'll be well on your way to health.

Self-Regulation	Structure & Mobility	Microbiome	Immune Balance	Angiogenic Balance	DNA Repair & Antioxidants	Regeneration & Autophagy	Detox & Excretion	Stress Mgmt.
	X	X	X	X	X	X		

X = the food is potentially harmful to the associated healing system

Fat is very calorie-dense, and sugar tends to make people overeat. When you combine fat and sugar, you are likely to eat way too many calories, and you will gain weight as a result.

A high-fat diet causes an increase in the bacteria that thrive off fat. Then, those fat-loving bacteria send signals to your brain to make you crave more fat.

High-heat meat processing generates advanced glycation end products (AGEs), which contribute to inflammation and premature aging.[240]

Sweet, saturated fats damage your blood vessels and inhibit angiogenesis, thus limiting your ability to heal tissues and fight off disease.[241]

Fatty foods (a.k.a. sweet saturated fat) may epigenetically change your predisposition to gain weight.[242] When you eat more sweet fats, you turn on the genes that tell your body to store calories rather than burn them off.

Meat isn't "sweet" per se, but there is often added sugar and sodium in processed meat. Studies show that processed meat is associated with oxidative stress, DNA damage, and telomere shortening.[243] [244] One MESA study showed that processed meat was the *only* food that could shorten telomeres.[245]

People with diets high in saturated fat have impaired abilities to activate and mobilize stem cells, especially in the brain.[246] [247]

Sweet, saturated fats damage endothelial stem cells and hurt your blood vessels. However, sweet fats don't impair the stem cells that regenerate your fatty tissue.[248] In effect, you will continue to get fatter while your body gets worse at healing itself.

Habit Hacks:

- The most effective way to stop eating junk food is to simply not buy it. When it's not in your home, you won't have to rely on willpower all the time, and you won't eat as much. So, on your future grocery escapades, don't shop hungry, only shop the perimeters of the store, or have someone else shop for you.

- If you have processed junk in your house, put it on the top shelf, in the back of the fridge, or in a place that is difficult to access. That way, you'll increase the number of steps it takes to consume processed food, and it'll be easier to break that bad habit.

- Post your grocery receipt on social media. If you buy junk food, tell people to call you out on it. Making bad habits public and painful will help you break the habit.

Tips & Tricks:

- Buy unsweetened products and add sugar to taste. It is okay to add sugar because you probably won't over-sweeten as much as the processed food manufacturers. Even so-called healthy brands will over-sweeten their products because "sweet sells."

- If you're going to add sugar to a meal, use honey. It is harder to spoon honey onto your food, and it doesn't dissolve as readily as sugar, so you probably won't eat as much.

- If a food comes with a barcode and colorful packaging, it's probably a Frankenfood. If it has a label like "lowers cholesterol" or "low sugar," there are probably some weird chemistry experiments going on behind the scenes. Remember, marketers are trying to persuade you to buy their product. A carrot, on the other hand, doesn't need to tell you that it's healthy.

- Only buy what your great-grandma could make in her kitchen. Could those crackers in your hand be made in a kitchen? Probably not. Most processed foods come from a laboratory, not an oven.

- Manufacturers often try to mask their sugar content by using five or six different types of sweeteners. That way, they can distribute the sugar content across five products rather than listing "sugar" as the number one ingredient. Some examples of artificial sweeteners include saccharin, aspartame, sucralose, acesulfame, and neotame.

- Before two years old, don't give your baby much gluten. Excess gluten as a baby increases the risk of developing celiac disease and gluten sensitivity.[249]

- If you'd like to know if you are at risk for gluten sensitivity, the DQ2 and DQ8 genes are associated with gluten intolerance.[250] This does not guarantee sensitivity, but you might wish to ask your doctor for a genetic test.

- The DPT4 enzyme may help you break down gluten and reduce its detrimental inflammatory effects. Maybe consider supplementing with this enzyme before you have a splurge day.

Step #3:

Drink Water

Water enables all life to exist. Considering that you, too, are alive, you probably want to put a lot of water in your body. Need I say more?

H_2O

Best of the best: the liquid form

Self-Regulation	Structure & Mobility	Microbiome	Immune Balance	Angiogenic Balance	DNA Repair & Antioxidants	Regeneration & Autophagy	Detox & Excretion	Stress Mgmt.
✔	✔	✔	✔	✔	✔	✔	✔	✔

✔ = the behavior is beneficial to the associated healing system

Every self-healing system requires water to function correctly. Therefore, I'm not going to repeat the same explanations every time; I'll just list a few.

👤 There are approximately 37 trillion cells in your body, and about 65% of every cell is water.[251] Your cells need water. Give it to them.

👤 Water allows your cells to transduce energy more effectively. The more hydrated you are, the more likely you'll feel energetic and youthful.

👤 Water helps you absorb and transport nutrients into your cells: more water = more nutrients.

🧍 Water in your joints and tissues allows your muscles and bones to glide and move smoothly, with fewer restrictions and adhesions. Also, your muscles are 70-75% water. In short, water helps your body feel and move like a young person.

☢ Water is our primary transport mechanism for toxins. The more water you consume, the better you are at detoxifying.

☢ Water makes you pee, and pee carries toxins out of your body. The more you pee, the more toxins you excrete, so drink more water!

Habit Hacks:

- Carry a water bottle with you all the time. When water is immediately available, you'll be reaching for it unconsciously and hydrating throughout the day.

- When trying to form a new habit, try stacking multiple habits on top of each other. If you already have a routine set of habits that you perform every day, squeeze in your new habit amongst the rest (like a habit sandwich). For example, when you wake up in the morning, after brushing your teeth, drink one full glass of water while your coffee is brewing. Here, you have stacked three habits on top of each other: brushing your teeth, drinking water, and drinking coffee. Plus, this habit uses temptation bundling by pairing a habit you want to do (drink coffee) with a habit you need to do (drink water). These strategies will make your water-drinking habit easier to complete every day.

- Get one of those hydration apps so you can track how much water you drink each day. Tracking your habits makes it easier to uphold a routine. Then, when you hit your goal for the day, give yourself a small reward. A reasonable goal is to drink at least 1/2 your body weight in ounces of water.

Tips & Tricks:

- Your brain often confuses thirst with hunger. When you feel hungry, you probably need water more than you need food.

- If your pee is darker yellow, you are dehydrated. Your goal is to have light yellow or clear pee and use the bathroom about once every two hours.

- Get a filter for your municipal tap water. I'm not a staunch follower of this rule, but it's probably a good idea.

Other Beverages

I still think that water is all you need, but I admit that some beverages carry incredible benefits. For those of you who just can't drink water all day, every day, try these drinks in addition to your daily water requirements.
P.S. When I say coffee, I mean brewed coffee. Those frappe mocha cappuccino concoctions are not coffee; they are sugar in a cup.

Best of the best: Red wine (1-2 glasses/day maximum), Tea (green/mint/black/oolong/chamomile), Coffee (not after 12pm)

	Self-Regulation	Structure & Mobility	Microbiome	Immune Balance	Angiogenic Balance	DNA Repair & Antioxidants	Regeneration & Autophagy	Detox & Excretion	Stress Mgmt.
Red Wine			✔	✔	✔		✔	✔	
Tea		✔	✔	✔	✔	✔	✔	✔	✔
Coffee	✔			✔	✔	✔		✔	

✔ = the behavior is beneficial to the associated healing system

Coffee stimulates BDNF production, which helps you form new nerve connections in your brain.[252]

Green tea may help maintain bone density.[253]

Coffee and tea (green, oolong, or black) can balance your microbiome by stimulating healthy bacteria and reducing bad bacteria.[254]

Red wine is food for good bacteria (prebiotic) via resveratrol and polyphenols.[255] [256]

Kombucha is a fermented tea made from a bacterial starter, called a SCOBY. Therefore, by drinking kombucha, you get a bunch of good bacteria.

✳ Green tea has vitamin C, which increases the production of T-regulatory cells.[257] Therefore, green tea helps restore balance in your immune system and turns down inflammation at the right times.

✳ Coffee and black tea are anti-inflammatory due to chlorogenic acid.[258] Red wine is, too, due to its abundance of polyphenols.[259]

◇ Red wine and beer can be antiangiogenic and improve blood vessel flexibility. Drink less than two glasses per day, though; any more produces the reverse effect.[260] [261]

◇ Coffee and tea (earl grey, jasmine, green, black chamomile, and sencha) help balance angiogenesis, reduce blood pressure, and improve vascular health.[262] [263]

✖ Coffee and tea turn on tumor suppressor genes to help you fight off tiny tumors before they grow into a problem.[264] [265]

✖ One cup of black coffee per day can slow aging by lengthening your telomeres.[266] [267] Tea drinking is associated with increased telomere length, too.[268]

↻ Red wine increases the circulation of endothelial progenitor cells and activates stem cells that usually lie dormant in the heart.[269] Thus, red wine can be good for your blood vessel and heart health. Too much red wine, though, is damaging to stem cells.

↻ Green and black tea activate stem cells to promote wound healing[270] and improve brain[271], muscle[272], and bone health[273] (via catechins).

↻ Chlorogenic Acid in coffee and black tea improves stem cell survival by making the stem cells more resilient to stress. At the same time, it helps kill lousy stem cells.[274]

☢ Coffee and coffee fruit contain antioxidants,[275] and wine helps you absorb more antioxidants from your healthy diet.[276] [277]

☢ Green tea epigenetically activates the genes responsible for producing glutathione, thus protecting your DNA from free radicals.[278]

☯ Green and black tea increase dopamine, serotonin, and glycine levels (via L-theanine). Glycine helps calm your brain while dopamine and serotonin make you feel good. These teas also induce alpha-brain wave activity, which is a characteristic of being in a relaxation state.[279] [280] [281]

LIMIT ALCOHOL & SUGARY BEVERAGES

Self-Regulation	Structure & Mobility	Microbiome	Immune Balance	Angiogenic Balance	DNA Repair & Antioxidants	Regeneration & Autophagy	Detox & Excretion	Stress Mgmt.
✗	✗	✗	✗	✗	✗	✗	✗	✗

✗ = the behavior is potentially harmful to the associated healing system

- Sugary drinks are at the bottom of the totem pole when it comes to food quality. Sugary drinks provide a lot of calories but virtually zero nutrients.

- The way you feel during a hangover is basically how your cells feel. Alcohol destroys your body's ability to work effectively.

- Alcohol does not help you fall asleep faster; it just sedates your brain and knocks you unconscious sooner. Alcohol makes your sleep more fragmented and blocks your REM sleep. So, you wake up feeling unrefreshed and unrestored.

- "Reducing sugar-sweetened beverage consumption may be the single best opportunity to curb the obesity epidemic." [282] Sodas and juices aren't the only culprits, either. Most alcoholic drinks are just liquid sugar, hard alcohol included.

- Alcohol promotes the growth of infectious gram-negative bacteria and increases intestinal permeability (via accumulation of acetyl aldehyde and nitrous oxide). [283] [284]

- Alcohol is a known immunosuppressor. The more you drink, you increase your risk for infections, inflammation, and disease. [285]

- Drinking sugar-sweetened beverages is associated with increased CRP levels, a marker for excessive inflammation in your body. [286]

- Alcohol promotes angiogenesis in excess, which allows tumors to commandeer a blood supply and develop into cancer. [287]

- High concentrations of glucose and fructose within sugary beverages contribute to angiogenic dysfunction. [288]

Excess alcohol consumption reduces the production of an enzyme called SAM. SAM helps epigenetically turn DNA on and off. Without SAM, your DNA may turn on at inappropriate times and contribute to aging and disease in the long run.[289]

Heavy drinking kills stem cells and hinders the function of stem cells in the memory center of your brain, the hippocampus.[290] When binge drinking stops, the damage reverses.

Alcohol is very demanding on your body. When your liver detoxifies alcohol, it must devote all its attention to the alcohol; it cannot simultaneously detoxify any other toxins. Fructose has this same effect. So, if you have alcohol AND fructose (aka mixed drinks or hard liquor), you are doing double damage.

Alcohol is highly toxic to your kidneys and brain, too.

"Phew, I need a drink." This common phrase represents how stress often triggers alcohol consumption. And even though having a drink with loved ones can reduce your stress, alcohol is not a stress-reliever. Socializing and bonding is the true hero; alcohol is just a useless sidekick that we bring along for no good reason.

Habit Hacks:

- Reframe your mindset. Instead of worrying about the sacrifices associated with cutting down on alcohol and sugary beverages, focus on the benefits you will gain. If you need some motivational ammunition, might I recommend the examples above?
- Remove the cues of your bad habit from your environment. For example, seeing a beer in your fridge may be a cue that you "need a beer," so take the beers out of the fridge. You can keep drinks in the house for your friends but consider putting them in an obscure location or behind a locked door.

Tips & Tricks:

- Sweet drinks are desserts; treat them as such. The only beverage you should be regularly consuming is 100% H_2O. Don't drink your sugar.
- If you must drink, choose dry, organic red wine. Only drink 1-2 glasses per day and never drink alone. And no, you can't save up for the weekend and drink ten glasses at once.
- Swap out your alcoholic or sugary beverage with water, red wine, tea, or coffee. Put it in an opaque cup and see if anyone notices. Or be straightforward and see if anyone cares. Besides giving you a bit of a hard time, I doubt you'll lose any friends over this.

STEP #4:

SLEEP LIKE YOU MEAN IT

Every animal sleeps. So, for 1/3 of the day, every animal is willing to give up eating, mating, and watching out for predators.

Why do we make such costly sacrifices to sleep? Because quality sleep is like the Swiss Army knife of health behaviors. By getting better sleep, you can improve nearly every system in your body. Conversely, if you struggle with an illness or other ailment, poor sleep is likely a contributor.

Also, consider this fun fact. When we lose one hour of sleep in the springtime due to daylight savings, there's a 24% increase in heart attacks, car accidents, and suicide rates. When we gain an hour of sleep in the fall, heart attacks decline by 21% the next day.[291]

SLEEP

Best of the best: the restful kind

Self-Regulation	Structure & Mobility	Microbiome	Immune Balance	Angiogenic Balance	DNA Repair & Antioxidants	Regeneration & Autophagy	Detox & Excretion	Stress Mgmt.
✔	✔		✔		✔	✔	✔	✔

✔ = the behavior is beneficial to the associated healing system

Sleep does terrific things for memory and learning. In the last two hours of sleep, your brain presses the save button on the things you learned throughout the day. Then, like wringing out a sponge, sleep cleanses your learning palate and prepares you to soak in more information tomorrow. Also, compared to getting no sleep, sleeping for more than 8 hours per night doubles the number of neural connections in your brain. Call me crazy, but I'd say that sleep literally makes you smarter.[292] [293]

The phrase, "You can sleep when you're dead" is meant to motivate productivity. But, as it turns out, the opposite is true. High-quality sleep makes you more productive, while poor sleep decreases productivity and increases all-cause mortality.[294] [295] So, without proper sleep, you'll die sooner, get sick more often, and be worthless throughout the day.

Your brain is affected by sleep more than any other system. Poor sleep is one of the most significant contributors to Alzheimer's disease.

Men who sleep 5-6 hours per night have the testosterone levels of a man who is ten years older.[296] [297] These underslept men also have smaller testicles, produce fewer sperm, and their sperm have more deformities and less motility.[298] If you want a better sex life, or if you're trying to have a baby, sleep more.

Poor sleep messes up your hormones to promote weight gain. When you are sleep deprived, you produce more ghrelin and less leptin, making you hungrier and prone to overeating.[299] Sleep deprivation also raises cortisol levels, which stimulates fat production.[300]

There is scientific proof that the more you sleep, the more attractive you appear.[301] [302] A.k.a. we've proven that beauty sleep is real.

Sleep alters muscle memory and increases peak force in muscles, which leads to improved reaction times, reduced injury rates, increased accuracy and speed, and decreased fatigue.[303] In other words, your brain is practicing while you sleep! If you want to be a better athlete, artist, employee, etc., sleep like you mean it.

Your immune system is most active while you sleep. After one night of inadequate sleep (<4 hours), natural killer cell activity decreases by 70%.[304] One night! Since natural killer cells play an essential role in stopping cancer and tumor growth, we could reasonably assume that lack of sleep increases your risk for cancer and tumors. That is why working the night shift is now considered a carcinogen.

Lack of sleep also stimulates unnecessary inflammation.[305]

Sleep regulates upwards of 15% of your genes. A single night of sleep deprivation can interfere with as many as 269 genes, including tumor-promoting genes[306] and the genes associated with fat metabolism, thus making you prone to obesity.[307]

Cell recycling and healing occur while you sleep. If you are not sleeping well, you are not healing well.

When you sleep, your glymphatic system kicks into gear, and power washes your brain. Namely, the glymphatic system helps clean out the amyloid plaques associated with Alzheimer's disease.[308]

Poor detoxification and poor sleep are intimately related. If you want to do a 'detox cleanse,' restful sleep must be a priority.

Restful sleep puts your body in a more relaxed, creative, and insightful state.[309] [310] Contrarily, poor sleep keeps your cortisol levels elevated and limits your ability to cope with stress.

Sleep is the ultimate antidepressant. One full night of sleep raised depression scores by 6 points on the Harrington Depression Scale, while the most effective antidepressants only improved depression scores by 1.5 points.[311] Similarly, most suicides occur when someone is sleep-deprived.[312]

Picture a young kid having a temper tantrum in the grocery store. The kid's parents will often say, "I'm sorry; he/she didn't sleep well last night." Those parents are correct; poor sleep (specifically, a lack of REM sleep) is associated with poor emotional regulation. And adults are just as likely to be emotionally affected by poor sleep. But, instead of a public outburst, our "tantrum" might show up as misplaced anger, frustration, impulsivity, or a general lack of emotional control. When you get high-quality REM sleep, though, you recalibrate the emotional centers in your brain. Sleep is like an emotional first aid.

Habit Hacks:

- Regularity is one of the most important factors for quality sleep. Get in the habit of going to bed and waking up at the same time every day, even on weekends. To help form this habit, write down an easy activity that will at least get you started. For example, "At 10:00 pm, I will have my pajamas on, and I will untuck the corner of my bedsheets." You technically don't *have* to go to bed, but you at least form the habit of being ready for bed at the same time every night.

- Create a bedtime ritual. Like shooting a free throw, having a consistent routine will prepare your brain for rest so that you will fall asleep easier. Try reading a book for 10-30 minutes or listen to an audiobook. Maybe pillow-talk with your significant other is a calming routine for you. Choose an activity that is not very "active." You want to wind down, not get riled up. To help form this habit, choose an activity that is very easy to complete. For example, use the two-minute rule.[313] Read for 2 minutes before going to bed. Seriously, after two minutes, stop reading. If you are enjoying the book, of course, you can continue, but as soon as you hit the point when it feels like work, just stop. You can use this strategy for any time-based habit. Downscaling the habit into shorter increments will make the habit more achievable and thus easier to ritualize.

Tips & Tricks:

- The ideal sleep schedule is around 10 pm to 6 am (because it aligns with the sun), but the best way to know if you are getting adequate sleep is to gauge how you feel. Do you wake up refreshed, without an alarm clock, and without needing caffeine? You can also take the MEQ test to help you determine if you're a morning person, a night owl, or somewhere in between.

- When the temperature of your room is a couple of degrees colder at night, you sleep better. The optimal sleeping temperature is 65°. Also, make sure your bedroom is completely dark. Any bit of light can reduce your sleep quality or wake you up unnecessarily.

- Shut your screens off at least one hour before bed. Blue light from electronic devices can switch off melatonin production and make it harder to fall asleep. Wind down with a book, meditation, or a creative activity instead. Alternatively, you can wear blue blocker glasses or turn on 'night-time' mode on your devices.

- No caffeine after noon. Caffeine blocks your production of adenosine (the sleepiness hormone). Adenosine accumulates throughout the day and peaks after 16 hours of wakefulness. If you drink caffeine after noon, your brain won't generate enough adenosine, and you won't be very sleepy at night.

- Try not to eat within three hours of going to bed. Eating causes blood to rush to your gut instead of your brain. But your brain needs lots of blood to run your glymphatic system (the cerebral power wash). So, at least once a week, prioritize sleep by eating early and getting quality rest.

- You don't sit around the dinner table waiting to get hungry, so don't sit in your bed waiting to get sleepy. If your mind is racing, spend less time in bed. You want your brain to associate the bed with sleep, not a wandering mind. Instead, sit or lay somewhere else in your house until you start getting sleepy again. Try meditating or taking your mind on a pleasant walk.

- Alcohol doesn't help you sleep better; it just sedates your brain. That's why people feel so tired after a night of drinking. Their sleep is fragmented and shallow, so they wake up feeling unrefreshed and unrestored, even if they slept over 10 hours.

STEP #5:

MOVE NATURALLY AND PLAY

Do you ever dread going to the gym? Yea, me too, because working out *feels* like work; there's no fun in it anymore. But it doesn't have to be that way.

If you are like most people, you aren't trying to be a pro athlete or an Olympic powerlifter. Instead, your goal is to be fit enough to do the activities you enjoy for the rest of your life. And thankfully, you can achieve this goal *and* have fun along the way; you don't have to suffer through the same old workout routine.

Also, being a "mover" is more important than being an "exerciser." If you have an active lifestyle that keeps you moving for most of the day, you'll look and feel better than the desk worker who needs to spend two hours at the gym. The longest-living people on Earth rarely go to the gym, but they stay fit and healthy because their lifestyle is a constant expression of movement and exercise.[314]

Granted, weight-training is a useful tool — the WHO recommends at least two days of weight training per week. But lifting weights doesn't have to be a sterile, lifeless routine of sets and reps. If you enjoy weightlifting, be my guest. But if not, there are plenty of other ways to make exercise fun and challenging at the same time.

Consider this. When you go for a walk with friends or family, you can make it fun by playing around with different ways to move. You can climb trees, hop from stone to stone, or forage for edible plants. While out biking, rollerblading, or running, you can enjoy the changing seasons and the new scenery each day. Your brain will literally light up with happiness chemicals when you engage and play in your natural environment. Even while you are working, you can play around with different body positions at your desk. You can stand, kneel, or sit cross-legged instead of adopting one seated position all day.

Being an "adult" and having "responsibilities" does not mean you have to stop playing, imagining, and exploring. These qualities are what make our species successful. For example, an artist creates masterpieces by playing around with different brush strokes, color palettes, and ideas. Companies like Apple continue to create innovative products because they play, tinker, and fiddle around with their designs. In the words of Todd Hargrove, "Play is not about doing things that are immature, frivolous, or trivial. It is about getting absorbed in an activity that is intrinsically motivating."[315]

Play means you practice and fiddle around with different ways of doing things until it falls into place. You tinker and fine-tune until it feels right.

So, whether you are at the gym or out in nature, play around with your movements. By tinkering and fine-tuning, you'll start to enjoy exercise because your workout routine will look less like work and routine. Pretty soon, you'll be craving activity, and fitness will just come naturally.

MOVEMENT & PLAY

Best of the best: the kind that you enjoy

SELF-REGULATION	STRUCTURE & MOBILITY	MICROBIOME	IMMUNE BALANCE	ANGIOGENIC BALANCE	DNA REPAIR & ANTIOXIDANTS	REGENERATION & AUTOPHAGY	DETOX & EXCRETION	STRESS MGMT.
✔	✔	✔	✔	✔	✔	✔	✔	✔

✔ = the behavior is beneficial to the associated healing system

👤 Exercise increases the volume of neurons in your brain and helps you improve your capacity to learn new skills and obtain memories. For example, after age 45, your hippocampus shrinks by 1-2% per year. Exercise has been shown to prevent this decline.[316]

👤 Play rewires the brain to enhance your social-emotional skills, cognitive and memory abilities, psychomotor skills, and self-regulation capacities. Therefore, play will help improve your relationships, productivity, and adaptability to stress, which sets the foundation for your future health.[317]

🧍 Immobility is the equivalent of rust on a car. If you let your body sit around, not doing anything, your muscles will atrophy, your bones will weaken, your arteries will clog, and your joints will degenerate. Meanwhile, exercise builds muscle mass, lessens fatty infiltration, and strengthens bones. If you want to move better, move more.

🪲 The short-chain fatty acid, butyrate, increases with exercise. Butyrate feeds your good bacteria and fortifies your gut wall.[318]

❋ Exercise enhances immune function and limits unnecessary inflammation. Merely moving your muscles helps push lymph through your body so you can clear away the dead and unwanted material that may build up in your tissues.

◈ After a hard workout, your body turns on angiogenesis to bring more nutrients to your muscles.[319]

✖ Exercise protects your DNA from damage and prevents telomere shortening.[320] Better yet, walking for 60 minutes per day lengthens telomeres and may increase your life by up to 25 years![321]

↻ Exercise stimulates cellular recycling and rejuvenation (aka autophagy).[322] [323]

↻ Brisk walking encourages regeneration, growth, and rewiring of neurons (via IGF-1 and BDNF).[324] It also increases blood flow to your brain, making you more creative, resourceful, and intelligent.[325]

♠ Exercise amplifies the function of antioxidants.[326] Yoga, in particular, increases your levels of glutathione.[327]

♠ Sweating carries toxins out of your body, so bring on the heat!

☾ Exercise reduces anxiety and improves sleep quality.[328] [329] If you exercise less than two hours before bed, though, you may have a difficult time falling asleep due to the epinephrine and cortisol spike.

☾ Fitness is defined as the ability to survive and adapt to different conditions. By playing with your movements, you expose yourself to many unique scenarios and become more adaptable to those circumstances. In other words, you become more resilient to stress.

Side note: Movement Games

In the back of this book, you'll find a 'Movement Games' addendum, which has descriptions of various movement-based games that you can play by yourself or with a friend. By playing movement games, you will get more longevity and health benefits than weightlifting. Plus, it's way more fun than the monotonous chore of lifting heavy things ten times and putting them down again.

Habit Hacks:

- Change your environment to prioritize movement and play over lounging around. For example, push your couch far away from the TV and put a mat on the ground instead. You are more likely to sit on the floor and practice mobility if you have space for it. While watching TV, you can play around with different positions and stretches, which is great for movement health and long-term mobility. Also, getting up and down off the floor is a great predictor of longevity.

- Make sports equipment, exercise equipment, toys, and games easily accessible. When exercise is more convenient, you are more likely to do it. Meanwhile, make sedentary activities less accessible and out of sight. Consider putting your TV behind cabinet doors and hiding the remote. Every extra step you add will make your bad habit more inconvenient, and you'll be less likely to consume it.

- Use gateway habits. Instead of saying, "I will go for a run every day," say, "I will put on my running shoes at x:xx o'clock every day." Smaller habits are less ominous, so you are more likely to maintain them.

- Use the two-minute rule — downscale your habit into a two-minute time frame. Once the two minutes are up, you are done for the day. If you want to keep going, you are welcome to, but you don't have to. Never miss twice, though. If you miss one day, make sure you keep the habit alive tomorrow.

- Create a motivation sandwich. Prepare for a difficult exercise by doing something you enjoy immediately beforehand. Then, after the exercise, cap it off with another enjoyable activity.

- Join a club, exercise group, or sports league. Creating a culture around your desired behavior helps you stay motivated.

- Use a habit tracker. Keep track of your habit streak, and don't break the daily chain. I like to use good ole' pencil and paper because physically writing a checkmark next to the habit gives me a sense of accomplishment.

Tips & Tricks:

- At your desk, alternate from sitting, standing, or walking (e.g., treadmill desk). Try to change positions every 15-30 minutes.

- Feeling antsy and overwhelmed is your body telling you to move more. Consider getting up and going for a walk.

- Every month or so, check in on your body's mobility and range of motion. Doing so will help you identify and fix any movement shortcomings that you may have developed. As a result, you'll be less likely to get injured, and you'll maintain your youthfulness for longer. The 'Mobility Check-Up' addendum in the back of the book will help guide you through this regular movement practice.

Activity Guidelines for Lifelong Youth

Guideline	Description	Examples
5x/wk or 150min/wk Move and be active (moderate physical activity):	Moderate activities feel like work, but not in an unpleasant way. Your heart rate is elevated to a point where it would be challenging to sing but easy to talk (60-80% of your max heart rate).	Brisk walking/Hiking Gardening/Yardwork Household chores Jogging Cycling/Mountain biking Swimming Playing around (e.g., climb, swing, chase, jump, crawl)
1-2x/wk Do something heavy	Whether you do these lifts in a gym or outdoors, make sure you expose yourself to all types of movements, not just one or two. Focus on proper form. Quality and control matter more than sets and reps. And remember, have fun! Play around with different movements and make it a game or competition.	Overhead push (e.g., chest/shoulder press) Overhead Pull (e.g., pull up, cable pull-down) Horizontal Push (e.g., push up, bench press) Horizontal Pull (e.g., rows) Squats Hip Hinge (e.g., deadlift) Lunges
1x/wk 20 minutes Do something vigorous to max out your heart rate	Vigorous activity feels hard and requires willpower to continue. Your breathing rate is high enough that you cannot have a conversation.	Sprint a hill five times HIIT Workouts Sprint Rowing Sprint biking Lap swimming for speed
Periodically Practice coordination, balance, and ROM	Focus on a movement that you are not very good at and do those movements more often. After all, you are only as strong as your weakest link.	Ankle mobility exercises Walk on an unstable surface (e.g., slackline, 2x4, curb) Yoga Play sports

STEP #6:

FIND YOUR TRIBE

Now that you have permission to play like a kid again, with whom are you going to play? Your friends, of course!

Unfortunately, in our busy culture, making time for friends is often neglected. But it should be a priority because socializing is one of the most dependable means of improving your health and happiness. The happiest people on Earth socialize at least eight hours a day, and the world's longest-living cultures spend much of their after-work time in a social setting.[330] [331]

However, when you hang out with your friends, try to do healthy activities. Instead of drinking and sitting around a table, you might choose to do movement-based activities like hiking or playing yard games. Behaviors are contagious, so if you choose to move, play, and socialize all at the same time, everyone will maximize their health and take another step toward Lifelong Youth.

CLOSE FRIENDS

Best of the best: anyone you can play with, laugh with, cry with, and talk openly. Your friends don't have to meet all these criteria; we choose different friends for different roles in our lives. But it will be good for your mental and emotional health if all these needs are met by a solid group of friends and family.

SELF-REGULATION	STRUCTURE & MOBILITY	MICROBIOME	IMMUNE BALANCE	ANGIOGENIC BALANCE	DNA REPAIR & ANTIOXIDANTS	REGENERATION & AUTOPHAGY	DETOX & EXCRETION	STRESS MGMT.
✔	✔	✔	✔	✔				✔

✔ = the behavior is beneficial to the associated healing system

Social isolation kills. It makes you more susceptible to disease[332] and contributes to an early death.[333] Social isolation is also associated with increased blood pressure.[334]

Choose your friends wisely. Your health will impact each other significantly. If your closest friends are obese, you are 57-71% more likely to be obese. And if your family members are obese, you are 40 times more likely to suffer the same fate.[335]

In the same way that people transfer diseases to each other, you also can share good bacteria by hugging, shaking hands, kissing, and being close to each other. Some people might be germophobic about this fact. You, however, should welcome it because it helps shape your microbiome.[336]

Social isolation is associated with increased C-reactive protein, a marker for inflammation.[337]

Socially isolated young adults exhibited slower wound healing and inadequate sleep quality.[338] This effect is primarily due to the stress of social isolation.

Friends make us laugh, help us through hard times, and support our endeavors. These are qualities that serve as an outlet for stress and make you more resilient to future stressors.

Habit Hacks:

- Join a club that meets regularly. Some people need a little nudge to hang out with friends, and it helps to have a scheduled time in their calendar.   .

Tips & Tricks

- Greet your friends and family in three ways: touch (e.g., hug), words of affirmation, and eye contact. This practice helps builds the relationship immensely and establishes a deeper connection.
- Find the healthiest person that you can stand and hang out with them as much as possible. Their health will rub off on you.
- An important determinant of happiness in the workplace is whether you have a best friend in the office. If you feel like your job is kind of a dud, make an extra effort to find a work buddy before you jump ship.
- Answer these questions to determine the quality of your friendships and their impact on your health.[339] Or use it to determine your individual qualities as a friend.
  - Do your friends smoke?
  - Are your friends overweight because of unhealthy behaviors?
  - Do they drink more than two glasses of alcohol per day?
  - Do they eat an unhealthy diet?
  - Are they excited about life, or are they prone to complaints and negativity?
  - Does their idea of recreation include watching TV and sitting around, or would they prefer to go outside and be active?
  - Are they curious about the world?
  - Do they listen as well as talk?
  - Are they interested in trying new things, or are they tied to a consistent routine?
  - Do they engage with the community and encourage your engagement?
  - Do you feel better or happier when you are around them?

Step #7:

Embrace Discomfort

There are two types of stress, psychological and physical. Psychological stress is emotional and mental; it makes you feel "stressed out" when you have a lot on your plate. People tend to get overwhelmed by psychological stress because it can last for a long time. We tend to worry about stressful events long after the event has ended, causing our stress level to persist unnecessarily. Meanwhile, physical stress comes from things that we physically do to our bodies, like lift weights, work under the hot sun, or sit in a sauna. Physical stress is what we are mostly referring to when we say things like "hard work pays off" and "what doesn't kill you makes you stronger."

But, in reality, a stressor is defined as anything that causes tension or strain. With this definition, I could say that just standing here is stressful. Gravity is pushing down on me, causing strain on my body, and I have to fight it to stay upright.

Gravity isn't bad for me, though, so how could I refer to it as stressful? Well, that's the moral of this chapter; not all stress is bad! Stress is really good for you; the problem is when we have too much stress, or it lasts for too long.

See, our bodies are like cups of coffee; they can only handle a certain amount of stress before they overflow. When you feel overwhelmed and anxious about all the things you need to get done, you've filled your cup up with too much psychological stress, and your anxiety is a sign that your cup is overflowing. But sometimes, your cup is filled up with just the right amount of stress. When you feel challenged, motivated, and eager to get to work, your job is probably providing the ideal amount of mental stress for you. Your daily tasks are likely just outside of your comfort zone, so the discomfort (a.k.a. stress) causes learning and growth rather than pain and anxiety. However, if your job is too easy (not enough stress), it won't challenge you to get better, and you'll feel bored and unmotivated.

Take exercise as another example. Exercise is stressful, and yet, we all know that exercise is good for us. But exercise is only good in the right amount. Too much exercise can be detrimental if you are not prepared for the stress. We see this often in the weekend warrior crowd. They sit around for most of the week and try to make up for their sedentarism with hard workouts and activities on the weekend.

Most of the time, these people end up getting injured. They didn't expose themselves to enough stress during the week, so their tissues were not prepared for the overload of stress once the weekend came around.

This is not to say that these people should stop doing the activities they enjoy; they just need to prepare appropriately. To stay young and injury-free, they need to build up their tissue tolerance throughout the week. Riding the rollercoaster of activity and inactivity is simply not going to work.

That brings up another good point; think of the stress that comes from riding a roller coaster. When you are on the ride for just a few minutes, all those stressful twists and turns are exhilarating and enjoyable. But imagine if you stayed on the roller coaster for three days straight. After a while, the stress of those twists and turns will become toxic rather than exciting. The same concept is true for psychological and physical stress. If you worry about your co-worker's derogatory comment for days after the event, your stress is probably doing more harm than good. Likewise, on mile three of your weekly run, you may be just fine. But if you decide to push on for longer than you have prepared for, you might be in some serious pain the next day.

In the end, it's all about finding the sweet spot. Too much stress for too long will overflow your cup and cause damaging effects in your body. Not enough stress will leave your body feeling frail, weak, vulnerable, or unmotivated. But if you have just the right amount of stress for just the right amount of time, your body will adapt by getting stronger and more resilient while feeling healthy and energized. In other words, appropriate stress management and finding the sweet spot for stress is the key to Lifelong Youth.

So, what is the threshold? How do you know when your cup will overflow? When do the beneficial effects of stress become negative?

I wish I could answer this question for you, but sadly I can't. Everybody has a different stress tolerance, and your tolerance level is always changing depending on your behaviors and environment.

Also, you might tolerate one type of stress quite well, but you struggle with other types. Maybe you are intolerant to the sun; you could get a sunburn on a cloudy day. But you are very tolerant of cold temperatures, and you could jump in a glacial lake without a shiver.

Thankfully, you can increase your tolerance to stress through training. This is called a specific adaptation to imposed demand, the SAID principle. Essentially, it means that if you want to build up your tolerance, you should incrementally expose yourself to more and more of that stress over time. Eventually, your body will get stronger and more resilient.

For fair-skinned people, you can use the SAID principle by sun-tanning. Tanning will train your skin cells to produce melanin, darkening your skin and making you more resilient to sunburn.

However, we all know that you can't just sit in the sun all day and expect a perfect bronzing. You have to build up your tan incrementally. If you try to do it all in one day, you won't be very happy tomorrow.

The same idea is true for any stressor. If you impose stress on yourself in a controlled, incremental way, you can increase your tolerance to that stress, thereby making you more resilient.

Again, this is all about finding the sweet spot between too much, too little, too long, or too short. To find your sweet spot, you have to play around with stress a little bit. Each time you expose yourself to controlled stress, pay attention to how your mind and body feels afterward. Could you have pushed a little harder in that workout yesterday, or did you go a little too hard, and you are sore for three days instead of one?

For some behaviors, it will be easy to see the results of too much or too little stress. When you get a sunburn, it is obvious that you stayed outside for too long. For most stressors, though, this is not the case. Your behaviors won't always give you immediate feedback.

So, as a general rule, lean into discomfort. Embrace it. Do things that are difficult, challenging, and a little bit uncomfortable. Your body likes to be challenged and pushed, and you are capable of more than you think. When you allow your body to adapt and grow, you'll be surprised how much progress you can make in a short amount of time.

Tips for embracing discomfort

You live in a world designed for constant comfort. Just think, you could spend your entire life inside climate-controlled buildings and weather-resistant cars if you had no reason to go outside. And if you wanted to, you could sit around all day, paying someone to do all your chores and heavy lifting.

Sometimes, it's okay to enjoy these comforts of human ingenuity; but there's a point when too much comfort means you aren't stressing yourself enough. By sitting in climate-controlled cars and houses all day long, you won't be prepared for physical stressors that require you to use your muscles or control your internal environment. Then, when a physical stressor inevitably arises, your unpreparedness is likely to result in injury or disease.

But if you embrace discomfort frequently, you will build up your resilience against all types of stress, and you'll be more prepared when an inevitable problem arises. Embracing discomfort trains your body to be stronger and more youthful, so you'll be less likely to get a disease and more likely to enjoy a happy and healthy life.

Use the tips below to help you embrace discomfort whenever you get the chance.

- Do things outside, in all types of weather. The easiest way to embrace discomfort is to step out of your climate-controlled box and experience the real world.

- Always be learning. Take a class, learn a skill, listen to podcasts, or read. People have spent years compiling their knowledge into a teachable form. By learning from others, you fill up a bank of knowledge that would have taken you many lifetimes to accumulate on your own. This bank of knowledge allows you to come up with creative solutions when difficult or stressful problems arise. The bigger your bank, the more prepared you will be to withstand the stress. So, keep learning!

- Do chores yourself, don't just hire someone to do it for you. For example, get up and vacuum your floor, don't rely on a robot to do your dirty work. At the very least, if you choose to outsource your chores, don't just sit around binge-watching Netflix. Use your freedom to challenge your mind and body. Learn and move!

- Get a coach or partner in crime. We usually underestimate how resilient we can be, and an accountability-buddy can help motivate you to do more than you thought possible.

- Track your thoughts and feelings after an activity. Was the activity mildly, moderately, or highly stressful? How long did the activity last? How did you feel during the activity? How do you feel afterward? For each activity that you want to track, create a table in a notebook, and answer these four questions every day. You'll be surprised how quickly you can determine your sweet spot of stress.

- View stress from a different perspective. Think of demanding tasks as challenges rather than threats. That way, you will no longer be the victim of stress but the master of it. Instead of just "dealing" with discomfort, you'll embrace it, welcome it, and seek it out.

On the following pages, I describe two unique examples of how a little discomfort can go a long way. Specifically, these examples focus on enduring uncomfortably hot and cold temperatures. In doing so, you trick your body into becoming more resilient, which has immense physiologic benefits for your long-term health.

COLD WATER IMMERSION

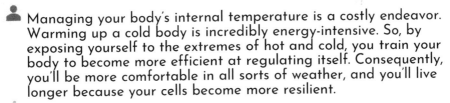

SELF-REGULATION	STRUCTURE & MOBILITY	MICROBIOME	IMMUNE BALANCE	ANGIOGENIC BALANCE	DNA REPAIR & ANTIOXIDANTS	REGENERATION & AUTOPHAGY	DETOX & EXCRETION	STRESS MGMT.
✓	✓	✓				✓		✓

✓ = the behavior is beneficial to the associated healing system

Managing your body's internal temperature is a costly endeavor. Warming up a cold body is incredibly energy-intensive. So, by exposing yourself to the extremes of hot and cold, you train your body to become more efficient at regulating itself. Consequently, you'll be more comfortable in all sorts of weather, and you'll live longer because your cells become more resilient.

Cold triggers adiponectin hormone production, which improves insulin sensitivity and increases your rate of fat loss.[340]

Exposure to cold stimulates the production of brown fat.[341] Brown fat is different from your typical white fat because instead of *storing* calories, brown fat will *burn* calories for energy, thereby helping you lose weight and improve your energy efficiency.

Your microbiome coats your skin with healthy oils, which protect your body and keep your skin looking vibrant and young. Hot showers will strip off these natural skin oils, but cold water keeps the oils intact.

When you jump into cold water, your body immediately enters 'protection-mode.' It thinks it needs to prepare for a long winter, so it will get rid of old and worn-out cells (a process called autophagy) and bring new and robust cells to the forefront. Essentially, you trick your body into becoming more resilient, and you are healthier as a result.

Cold exposure teaches you to calm your mind and body in stressful situations, which is a skill you can utilize in many aspects of life.

SAUNA

SELF-REGULATION	STRUCTURE & MOBILITY	MICROBIOME	IMMUNE BALANCE	ANGIOGENIC BALANCE	DNA REPAIR & ANTIOXIDANTS	REGENERATION & AUTOPHAGY	DETOX & EXCRETION	STRESS MGMT.
✔	✔		✔			✔	✔	

✔ = the behavior is beneficial to the associated healing system

👤 When you expose yourself to the hot and cold extremes, you get better at managing your internal body temperature. Therefore, you'll be able to withstand a wide range of temperatures, and you'll feel more youthful and resilient.

👤 Heat shock proteins produced during heat exposure (sauna) help prevent neurodegenerative diseases like Alzheimer's.[342]

🧍 Sauna is associated with increased levels of growth hormone.[343] Growth hormone helps build muscle and prevents atrophy. So, hop in the sauna after a workout to maximize your gains.

✳ Saunas stimulate your immune system by creating a rapid release of interleukin six (IL-6).[344]

🔄 Any heat that causes sweating (sauna, exercise, or a hot bath) may stimulate heat shock proteins.[345] These proteins tell your cells to buckle down, toughen up, and prepare for a scorching summer. Even though a hot summer is not actually approaching, your body doesn't know that. So, it gets rid of the old and weak cells to make room for new and robust cells. Consequently, your body gets more resilient and youthful. Thankfully, you only had to deal with 15 minutes in a sauna instead of a long, sweltering summer.

☢ Many water-soluble toxins leave your body via sweat. Since saunas make you sweat, you'll detoxify quicker.

Tips & Tricks:

- At the end of your shower, turn on the cold for 30 seconds. Yes, it will suck at first, but eventually, you may enjoy the cold. It will wake you up better than a cup of coffee, and you'll feel warmer when coming out of a cold shower (no more shivering under your towel).

- As an alternative to cold showers, put an ice pack on the back of your neck for 30 minutes every night. In adults, brown fat resides across your shoulders and down the spine. By placing an ice pack at the base of your neck, you will stimulate brown fat production. This strategy will not work as well as cold water immersion, but it is more tolerable for most people.

- If you have the luxury, go back and forth between a hot sauna and a cold shower or cold pool. This creates a kind of pumping effect in your blood vessels, which helps clear away toxins and debris.

- According to Wim Hof, you can control your body's response to cold by practicing a unique breathing technique called the Wim Hof Method. He has used this technique to perform amazing feats like climbing Mt. Everest without a shirt and swimming under the ice for 90 meters. So, before exposing yourself to cold water, consider trying his simple breathing tactics.

STEP #8:

PRACTICE SPIRITUALITY

You don't need to be religious to practice spirituality. No matter what you believe, the act of sharing your belief with others will add to your health and happiness. This is partly because spiritual gatherings help foster social ties. But spirituality also allows for quiet reflection and mindfulness, which relieves stress. I refer to spirituality as meditation and mindfulness in the following pages, but any faith system will likely have similar effects. You could substitute meditation and mindfulness with the words 'prayer' and 'reflection' if that is what makes you happy.

MEDITATION & MINDFULNESS

SELF-REGULATION	STRUCTURE & MOBILITY	MICROBIOME	IMMUNE BALANCE	ANGIOGENIC BALANCE	DNA REPAIR & ANTIOXIDANTS	REGENERATION & AUTOPHAGY	DETOX & EXCRETION	STRESS MGMT.
✔		✔	✔		✔	✔		✔

✔ = the behavior is beneficial to the associated healing system

Every time you focus your attention on something, your brain rewires itself by establishing new neural connections. With meditation and mindfulness, you often draw your attention toward positive emotions like kindness, love, and conscientiousness. In doing so, you literally reshape the structure of your brain. So, you aren't just 'faking it 'til you make it,' you *reshape it 'til you make it!*

Stress alters your microbiome, and since yoga and meditation can help mediate the effect of stress, they also improve microbial health.

Cortisol and stress dampen your immune system. Therefore, the stress-relieving effects of meditation can recalibrate your immunity.

Meditation lengthens telomeres by upregulating telomerase protein activity.[346]

Meditation also helps deactivate the genes associated with inflammation, which is implicated in almost every chronic disease that affects our aging population.[347]

Meditation increases stem cell count and improves their function.[348]

After a stress-triggering event, meditation, mindfulness, or quiet repose is one of the best ways to calm yourself down again. In other words, mindfulness helps empty your cup of stress so that it is less likely to overflow and cause damage.

Tips & Tricks

- Give your brain some downtime. Unplug for a little while every day, and don't do anything. Your brain's default mode is still active during this time, and it is working on problem-solving and creating new ideas. So, even if taking a break seems unproductive, you are more productive in the end.

- Stop multitasking; it's impossible. You are never actually doing two things at once; you are just quickly shifting your focus back and forth, which wastes time and energy. If you want to be more productive, focus on one job at a time.

- A standard breathing cadence for relaxation is to breathe in through your nose for five seconds, hold for seven seconds, and exhale for ten seconds through a relaxed jaw. Exhaling with a slow, long breath will stimulate parasympathetic activity and tell your body to rest, protect, and repair itself.

- Most people meditate by trying to focus as hard as they can on their breath, their mind's eyes, or some body part. But meditation is not meant to teach you how to focus; it is meant to teach you awareness. Your ability to focus may improve as a side-effect of meditation, but don't be frustrated if you get distracted during a session. Meditation is about acceptance, not judgment. So, whenever you lose focus, just tell yourself, "okay, I got distracted for a second; let's start again." Don't worry about perfection; just be present and aware of the way your mind works. We call it a meditation "practice" for a reason.

- My favorite meditation practice is inspired by Dan Siegel's Wheel of Awareness. I start by paying attention to each of my six senses (sounds, smells, tastes, the light coming through my eyelids, and the chair touching my body). Then, I scan my body, paying attention to my muscles and the sensations I feel over each body part. I end the session by thinking about all the things I am grateful for, and I must come up with one new or unique gratitude each time. If you prefer to explore a different type of meditation practice, try these other resources.
  - Wim Hof Method
  - Calm App
  - Headspace app

Conclusion:
The Full List

Congratulations! You've learned what it takes to live a long and youthful life. Now, it's time to turn your knowledge into action.

On the following pages, I have condensed the simple steps into a summary chart. You can print a copy of this chart by going to lifelongyouthbook.com/resources.

Then, you can hang the list on your fridge, bathroom mirror, or somewhere that you'll see it every day. Since these simple steps are not always easy to execute, it will be helpful to have a reminder that you can reference daily. You might also find it easier to stay motivated when you can plainly see all the reasons why your healthy behaviors are so good for you.

THE SIMPLE STEPS

Step #1: Find Your Sense of Purpose

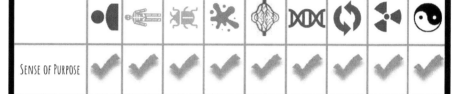

Step #2: Eat, Papa, Eat

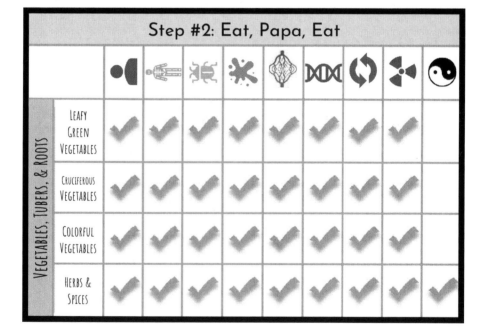

FRUIT									
Berries	✓		✓	✓	✓	✓	✓	✓	
Stone Fruit	✓		✓		✓	✓	✓		✓
Citrus Fruit	✓	✓	✓	✓		✓	✓	✓	
Other Fruit	✓	✓	✓	✓	✓	✓	✓	✓	

PRODUCTS FROM HEALTHY ANIMALS									
Muscle Meat	✓	✓			✓	✓		✓	
Organ Meat or Offal	✓	✓						✓	
Eggs	✓	✓		✓				✓	
Milk, Cheese, or Butter	✓	✓	✓		✓			✓	

Wild-Caught Seafood	✓	✓	✓	✓	✓	✓	✓	✓	✓
Nuts & Seeds	✓		✓	✓	✓	✓	✓	✓	
Legumes	✓		✓	✓	✓	✓	✓	✓	
Fungus	✓		✓	✓		✓	✓	✓	
Fermented Foods	✓		✓	✓	✓	✓	✓	✓	✓
Oils	✓	✓	✓	✓	✓	✓		✓	✓
Certain Grains	✓		✓	✓	✓	✓	✓		✓
EATING STRATEGIES — Fasting Mimicking	✓	✓	✓	✓	✓	✓	✓	✓	
EATING STRATEGIES — Time-Restricted Feeding	✓	✓	✓	✓	✓	✓	✓	✓	✓
EATING STRATEGIES — Ketosis Diet	✓	✓	✓	✓	✓	✓		✓	

FOODS TO LIMIT		1	2	3	4	5	6	7	8	9
	CORN	X	X	X						
	ARTIFICIAL SWEETENER, FRUCTOSE, & HIGH SUGAR	X	X	X	X		X	X	X	
	WHEAT FLOUR	X	X	X						
	"SWEET" SATURATED FATS		X	X	X	X	X	X		
	ALCOHOL	X	X	X	X	X	X	X	X	X

'Best of the Best' Food Examples

*Leafy Green Vegetables = kale, spinach, green/red leaf lettuce, dandelion, collard greens, endive, microgreens, swiss chard, leek, mustard greens
*Cruciferous Vegetables = broccoli, cauliflower, brussels sprouts, arugula, bok choy, cabbage, kohlrabi, radish, turnip, watercress, romanesco
*Colorful Vegetables = pepper, carrot, beet, sweet potato, squash, Chinese celery
*Stone Fruit = peach, plum, nectarine, lychee, apricot, cherry, mango, cacao
*Citrus Fruit = grapefruit, orange, guava, kiwifruit, pineapple
*Other Fruit = tomato, avocado, pomegranate, cranberry, grape, apple, eggplant, coconut (technically a tree nut), fig (technically a flower)
*Healthy Animal Products = wild game, organ meat (liver), bone broth, free-range chicken eggs, duck eggs, milk/cheese/butter from grass-fed cows
*Wild-caught Seafood = small fish (anchovies, sardines, herring), salmon, mackerel, other seafood (clams, oysters, mollusks, mussels)
*Nuts & Seeds = raw nuts (pistachio, macadamia, almond, hazelnut)
*Legumes = black beans, lentils, soy
*Fungus = porcini, white button mushrooms
*Fermented Foods = sauerkraut, kimchi, tempeh (soy), miso, natto, yogurt, kefir, kombucha, pickled veggies, vinegar
*Oil = extra virgin olive oil (EVOO), coconut oil, flaxseed oil
*Certain Grains = quinoa, oatmeal, sourdough, pumpernickel, rice bran

Step #3: Drink Water

	◗	🜨	🐢	✳	◈	DNA	↻	☢	☯
H₂O	✓	✓	✓	✓	✓	✓	✓	✓	✓
OTHER BEVERAGES — RED WINE			✓	✓	✓			✓	✓
OTHER BEVERAGES — TEA		✓	✓	✓	✓	✓	✓	✓	
OTHER BEVERAGES — COFFEE	✓		✓	✓	✓	✓	✓	✓	

Step #4: Sleep Like You Mean It

	◗	🜨	🐢	✳	◈	DNA	↻	☢	☯
QUALITY SLEEP	✓	✓		✓		✓	✓	✓	✓

Step #5: Move Naturally and Play

	◗	🜨	🐢	✳	◈	DNA	↻	☢	☯
MOVEMENT, EXERCISE, & PLAY	✓	✓	✓	✓	✓	✓	✓	✓	✓

Step #6: Find Your Tribe

	Self-Regulation	Structure & Mobility	Microbiome	Immune Balance	Angiogenic Balance	DNA Repair & Antioxidants	Regeneration & Autophagy	Detox & Excretion	Stress Mgmt.
Social Interaction	✓	✓	✓	✓	✓				✓

Step #7: Embrace Discomfort

	Self-Regulation	Structure & Mobility	Microbiome	Immune Balance	Angiogenic Balance	DNA Repair & Antioxidants	Regeneration & Autophagy	Detox & Excretion	Stress Mgmt.
Cold Water Immersion	✓	✓	✓				✓		✓
Sauna	✓	✓			✓	✓	✓	✓	

Step #8: Practice Spirituality

	Self-Regulation	Structure & Mobility	Microbiome	Immune Balance	Angiogenic Balance	DNA Repair & Antioxidants	Regeneration & Autophagy	Detox & Excretion	Stress Mgmt.
Meditation & Mindfulness	✓		✓	✓		✓	✓		✓

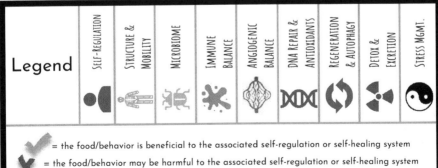

Legend — Self-Regulation, Structure & Mobility, Microbiome, Immune Balance, Angiogenic Balance, DNA Repair & Antioxidants, Regeneration & Autophagy, Detox & Excretion, Stress Mgmt.

✓ = the food/behavior is beneficial to the associated self-regulation or self-healing system

✗ = the food/behavior may be harmful to the associated self-regulation or self-healing system

The Simple Steps: Detailed List of Foods

The following list will give you some ideas about the common foods and behaviors that improve your self-healing and self-regulating systems. This list is extensive, and yet there are many things that I have not listed. Your job is to take this list and expand upon it. Explore new activities and try new flavors. With all the healthy options in the world, you could probably enjoy a new meal or activity every day of your life. So have fun with it. Soak up as much life as you can while you are still able. What's the point of Lifelong Youth if you don't enjoy the journey?

Foods:

The items in **Bold** are on the Lifelong Youth "**Best of the Best**" list.

Leafy Green Vegetables

Arugula
Beet leaves
Bibb lettuce
Chinese cabbage
Collard greens
Dandelion greens
Endive

Green leaf lettuce
Kale/Cavolo Nero
Leek
Microgreens
Mustard greens
Okra
Puha

Rapini
Red leaf lettuce
Romaine lettuce
Spinach
Swiss chard
Turnip greens
Witloof

Cruciferous Vegetables

Bok choy
Broccoli
Brussels sprouts
Cabbage

Cauliflower
Kohlrabi
Radish
Romanesco

Rutabaga
Turnip
Watercress

Colorful vegetables

Acorn squash
Artichoke
Asparagus
Bamboo shoots
Beets
Butternut squash
Carrots
Celery
Chayote squash
Chinese celery
Cucumber

Fiddleheads
Jicama
Onion
Parsnip
Peppers
Potato
Pumpkin
Purple potato
Radicchio
Rhubarb
Shallot

Spaghetti squash
Sprouts
Squash blossoms
Sweet pepper
Sweet potato
Taro
Winter squash
Yam
Yuca/cassava
Zucchini

Herbs & Spices

Aged garlic
Basil
Chile peppers
Cilantro
Cinnamon
Fennel
Garlic

Ginger
Ginseng
Licorice Root
Marjoram
Oregano
Peppermint
Rosemary

Saffron
Sage
Tahini
Thyme
Turmeric

Berries

Acai berry
Bearberry
Bilberry
Black currant
Black raspberry
Blackberry
Blueberry
Boysenberry
Capers
Chokeberry
Chokecherry

Cloudberry
Cowberry
Cranberry
Currant
Elderberry
Goji Berry
Gooseberry
Grape (concord)
Juneberry
Loganberry
Loquat

Lychee/soapberry
Mulberry
Persimmon
Raspberry
Salmonberry
Seaberry
Snowberry
Strawberry
Tayberry

Stone Fruit

Apricot
Barbados cherry
Breadfruit
Camu
Cherry

Coconut
Date
Lychee
Mango
Nectarine

Olive
Peach
Surinam Cherry
Plum
Pluot/Aprium

Citrus Fruit

Blood orange
Buddha's hand
Citron
Clementine
Grapefruit
Guava
Kiwifruit

Kumquat
Lemon
Lime
Mandarin
Orange
Orangelo
Papaya

Pineapple
Pomelo
Tangelo
Tangerine
Ugli fruit
Yuzu

Other Fruit

Apples	Fig	Quince
Avocado	Honeydew melon	Sapodilla
Banana	Horned melon	Sapote
Cacao	Jackfruit	Soursop
Cantaloupe	Java-Plum	Starfruit
Cherry tomato	Jujube fruit	Sugar-apple
Dark chocolate	Longan	Tamarind
Dragon fruit	Passion Fruit	**Tomatoes**
Durian	Pear	Tomatillo
Eggplant	Plantain	**Watermelon**
Feijoa	**Pomegranate**	

Animal meat from healthy animals or wild game

Beef	Goat meat	Pork/Ham
Chicken (dark)	**Pheasant**	Bison
Deer/venison	Turkey meat	Goose
Duck meat	Lamb	Quail

Organ meat/Offal from healthy animals

Beef liver	Elk	Haggis
Black pudding	Galbi	Suet
Chicken liver	Giblets	Sweetbread
Chitterlings	Gizzard	Tripe

Other animal products from healthy animals

Bone broth	**Goat butter**	**Grass-fed milk**
Camembert cheese	**Goat cheese**	Jarlsberg cheese
Chicken eggs	**Goat milk**	Muenster cheese
Duck eggs	Gouda	**Parmigiano**
Edam cheese	**Grass-fed butter**	**Reggiano**
Emmenthal cheese	**Grass-fed cheese**	Stilton cheese

Wild-caught/Sustainably raised seafood

Anchovies
Arctic char
Big eye tuna
Black bass
Bluefin tuna
Bluefish
Bottarga
Catfish
Caviar (sturgeon)
Clams
Cockles
Cod
Crawfish
Flounder
Grey mullet
Grouper

Haddock
Hake
Halibut
Herring
Lingcod
Mackerel
Mahimahi
Marlin
Mollusks
Mussels
Octopus
Oysters
Perch
Pollock
Pompano
Rainbow trout

Red mullet
Salmon
Sardines
Scallops
Sea bass
Sea bream
Sea cucumber
Seatrout
Shrimp
Snapper
Spiny lobster
Squid
Tilapia
Walleye
Yellowtail

If you are concerned about over-fishing, use this list of sustainable seafood from the Environmental Defense Fund: http://seafood.edf.org/

Nuts & Seeds

Almonds
Brazil nuts
Cashews
Chestnuts
Chia seeds
Hazelnuts

Macadamias
Peanuts
Pecans
Pine nuts
Pistachios
Pumpkin Seeds

Sesame seeds
Squash seeds
Sunflower seeds
Walnuts

Legumes

Black beans
Chickpeas
Green beans
Kidney beans
Lentils

Mung beans
Navy beans
Peas
Pinto beans
Snap peas

Snow peas
Soybeans
String beans

Mushrooms/Fungus

Black truffles
Black trumpets
White Button
Chanterelles

Enoki
Lion's mane
Maitake
Morel

Oyster mushrooms
Porcini
Portobello
Shiitake

Fermented Foods

Kefir	**Natto**	**Tempeh**
Kimchi	**Pao Cai**	**Vinegar**
Kombucha	**Pickled veggies**	**Yogurt**
Miso	**Sauerkraut**	

Oil

Coconut oil	**Extra virgin olive oil (EVOO)**	**Flaxseed oil**

Certain grains (whole grains, not flours)

Amaranth	Faro	**Quinoa**
Arrowroot	Flax	**Rice bran**
Barley	**Millet**	**Sourdough**
Buckwheat	**Oatmeal**	Wild rice
Einkorn wheat	**Pumpernickel**	

Beverages

Black tea	**Green tea**	Red wine
Chamomile tea	"Hoppy" beer	Sencha tea
Coffee (black)	Oolong tea	**Water**

The Simple Steps: Detailed List of Behaviors

This list of behaviors is small, but that does not mean your behaviors are less important than food. Actually, the list of healthy behaviors is infinite. There may be only one way to sleep, but there is no limit to the number of creative ways you can move, play, and socialize with others. So, don't let the size of this list confuse you; your behaviors are just as crucial to your health as your food choices.

Having a sense of purpose

Eating strategies
Fasting-mimicking diet
Time-restricted feeding
Ketosis diet

Quality sleep

Movement, exercise, & play
(see the 'Movement Games' addendum)

Social interaction

Embrace Discomfort
Cold water immersion
Sauna

Meditation & Mindfulness

ADDENDUM #1:

SPLURGE LIST

It's okay to splurge once in a while, but you don't have to go off the deep end just to "get your fix." And if you are going to splurge, why not splurge on foods that are better for your health yet still taste like you are getting away with something?

On the next page, you'll see the splurge chart. On the left side of the chart, there is a list of common splurge foods that are not-so-good for your health. On the right side, though, you'll find equally-as-tasty splurge food alternatives that are a bit better for your Lifelong Youth goals.

However, even though these are healthier alternatives, it does not mean you can eat them all the time. These foods are still considered splurge items, meant to be eaten as a special treat every month or so. Here's a rule of thumb: as soon as you stop getting excited about your splurges, you are probably doing it too much.

The best way to avoid too much splurging is to keep the splurge foods out of your house. Don't buy splurge foods on your regular shopping trip. Instead, wait until you get the urge to splurge. That way, your urges need to be significant enough to get you to walk, bike, or drive to a grocery store.

Otherwise, get the ingredients to make the splurge foods at home. That way, you'll need to do more than just open a cupboard door to soothe your cravings. Also, there are a lot of other benefits when making homemade goods. And homemade food typically has far less sugar, salt, and artificial additives compared to store-bought items. Plus, making the food yourself burns calories, and sharing your treat with others strengthens social ties. So, before you even eat the splurge food, you'll be combating it with the health benefits that come from making it yourself.

After your splurge session, don't beat yourself up about it. Your overall way of living matters more than an occasional misstep. If you are really worried, just make up for the splurge by eating healthy tomorrow. As long as it's not a frequent occurrence, your body will quickly recover from the indulgence, and you'll still be on the path to Lifelong Youth.

Splurge List

Trade the foods on the left ⇨ for the foods on the right

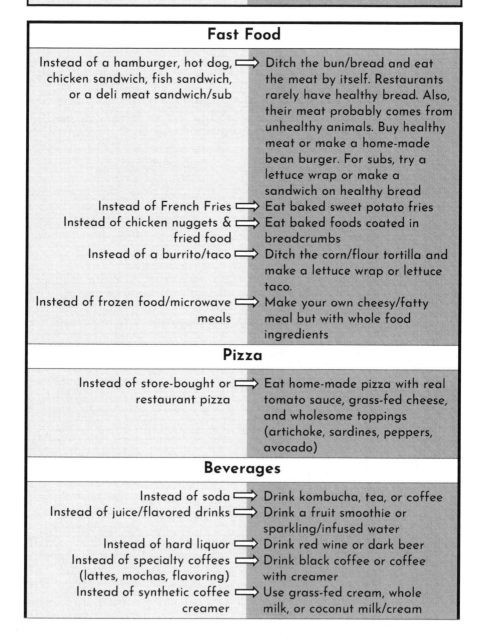

Fast Food

Instead of a hamburger, hot dog, ⇨ chicken sandwich, fish sandwich, or a deli meat sandwich/sub — Ditch the bun/bread and eat the meat by itself. Restaurants rarely have healthy bread. Also, their meat probably comes from unhealthy animals. Buy healthy meat or make a home-made bean burger. For subs, try a lettuce wrap or make a sandwich on healthy bread

Instead of French Fries ⇨ Eat baked sweet potato fries

Instead of chicken nuggets & ⇨ fried food — Eat baked foods coated in breadcrumbs

Instead of a burrito/taco ⇨ Ditch the corn/flour tortilla and make a lettuce wrap or lettuce taco.

Instead of frozen food/microwave ⇨ meals — Make your own cheesy/fatty meal but with whole food ingredients

Pizza

Instead of store-bought or ⇨ restaurant pizza — Eat home-made pizza with real tomato sauce, grass-fed cheese, and wholesome toppings (artichoke, sardines, peppers, avocado)

Beverages

Instead of soda ⇨ Drink kombucha, tea, or coffee

Instead of juice/flavored drinks ⇨ Drink a fruit smoothie or sparkling/infused water

Instead of hard liquor ⇨ Drink red wine or dark beer

Instead of specialty coffees ⇨ (lattes, mochas, flavoring) — Drink black coffee or coffee with creamer

Instead of synthetic coffee ⇨ creamer — Use grass-fed cream, whole milk, or coconut milk/cream

Candy

Instead of gummies ⟹ Eat dried fruit

Instead of hard candy ⟹ Eat frozen fruit (e.g., raspberries, grapes, mango)

Instead of caramels ⟹ Eat baked fruit (e.g., apples, peaches, nectarines)

Instead of milk chocolate ⟹ Eat chocolate with nuts or real peanut butter

Salty Snacks

Instead of chips ⟹ Eat home-made potato chips/sweet potato chips. Or eat crunchy veggies with dip or hummus (e.g., carrots, radishes, celery, snap peas, cucumbers & salt)

Instead of crackers ⟹ Eat pretzels and peanut butter or rice cakes

Instead of store-bought buttery popcorn ⟹ Buy bland popcorn and add your own grass-fed butter or coconut oil

Ice Cream

Instead of "airy/fluffy" ice cream (often branded as light, low fat, or low sugar). If you can take it out of the freezer and scoop it right away, it's probably emulsified b.s. ⟹ Eat organic ice cream from grass-fed cows (if unsure, get non-dairy versions) Or eat home-made ice cream with real cream and fresh fruit (if it comes out of the freezer and it is rock hard, it's probably made with real cream) Or eat home-made fruit popsicles

Instead of a fast-food shake ⟹ Eat a home-made smoothie made from real fruit (you can even add some sugar or dark chocolate)

Baked goods

Instead of packaged cake/donuts ⟹ Make a cake/donut from scratch

Instead of pie/cheesecake ⟹ Eat Greek yogurt with fruit

Instead of packaged cookies ⟹ Make cookies/ginger snaps from scratch

Breakfast Carbs

Instead of cereal/granola ⟹ Choose a "blander" cereal or eat oatmeal and add fruit (or just a little sugar)

Instead of a pop-tart/toaster strudel ⟹ Eat toast or a sourdough English muffin with egg/fruit/pb

Instead of waffles/pancakes ⟹ Eat home-made, low-sugar, or high fiber pancakes

Instead of muffins ⟹ Eat home-made flavored bread

Instead of fast-food hash browns ⟹ Eat home-made hash browns

Pasta & Bread

Instead of a spaghetti/pasta ⟹ Eat spaghetti squash or butternut squash

Instead of mac & cheese ⟹ Eat dairy-free or organic mac w/ grass-fed cheese

Instead of white bread, bagels, & tortillas ⟹ Eat sprouted bread that still has the "chunks" of grain/seed inside. Or make homemade sourdough

Instead of a fast-food breakfast sandwich/burrito ⟹ Eat an egg on a sourdough English muffin

Sports, Energy, or Protein Bars

Instead of store-bought energy/protein bars (which are generally unnecessary if you're not exercising regularly) ⟹ Eat home-made bars (e.g., oatmeal & PB or fruit & nut) Or eat trail mix Or eat hard-boiled eggs

Cooking Fats

Instead of butter substitutes ⟹ Use grass-fed butter, olive oil, coconut/avocado oil, or ghee

Condiments

Instead of sauces/dressing ⟹ Use olive oil, balsamic vinegar, lemon juice, soy sauce, s

Instead of ketchup or BBQ sauce ⟹ Use hot sauce or mustard

Instead of mayonnaise ⟹ Use grass-fed butter or home-made mayo

Instead of processed cheeses ⟹ Use cheese from grass-fed cows

Instead of processed syrup ⟹ Use pure maple syrup or fruit

Instead of jams/jellies ⟹ Use mashed fruit or full-fat peanut butter w/o added sugar

ADDENDUM #2:

COMMON TOXINS

Usually, your body is good at getting rid of toxins before they cause problems. But sometimes, it loses the battle. One reason is that some toxins are ubiquitous in our environment, and we are constantly exposed to them in our daily lives. With so much exposure, your body has a tough time getting rid of the toxin before it causes damage. Another reason is that the toxin is highly potent. Just a small dose of these substances can throw your whole body out of whack. In both instances, your best strategy against ubiquitous or highly potent toxins is to limit your exposure.

Therefore, in the upcoming pages, I describe some of the toxins that commonly appear in our environment. Below each toxin, I'll give you some examples of where these toxins are found and how you can limit your exposure.

Persistent organic pollutants (POPs) - this type of toxin is known as an obesogen because its presence in your blood is correlated with obesity. When you have more POPs in your system, you produce more visceral fat, which causes inflammation and reduced cellular function. These toxins are "persistent" because they continue to circulate in the environment, causing damage to animals and ecosystems.

- **Examples of POPs:**
  - o DDT pesticide, which is now banned in the USA.
  - o Polychlorinated biphenyls (PCBs) - found in plastics, fuels, and some paints.
  - o Dioxins - a byproduct of some types of manufacturing and fuel-burning.
- **Tips for limiting exposure:**
  - o Make your own household cleaners and disinfectants (water, baking soda, borax, essential oils, vinegar, hydrogen peroxide, and castile soap are all great ingredient choices).
  - o Avoid buying plastics, sunscreen, and sheets that contain POPs. Go to ewg.org for a list of consumer products that are healthy for your body and the environment.

Endocrine disruptors - these toxins look and act like your body's natural hormones. When they get into your body, they block your cell receptors and create a cascade of dysfunction within your cells, which may eventually lead to total organ malfunction. Some examples of endocrine disruptors are:

- **Fluoride, chlorine, and bromine** - typically found in municipal water systems. They act like thyroid hormones and may lead to symptoms of hypothyroidism because they block your thyroid receptors. Men with infertility issues might consider checking their blood for these substances.
  - o **Tips for limiting exposure:**
    - Install a chlorine filter on your showerhead.
    - Use fluoride-free toothpaste.
    - Limit your intake of food that is exposed to a lot of agricultural chemicals and insecticides. Google 'EWG Dirty Dozen' for a quick list of the nastiest food culprits.

- **Plastics (PCBs, BPA, BPL, & phthalates)** - these substances look and act like estrogen, so they add fat to your body as if you were preparing for an upcoming pregnancy (males included). They can also lead to congenital disabilities, breast cancer, testicular cancer, and infertility.[349] [350] [351]
  - o **Tips for limiting exposure:**
    - Vitamin B12, B9, choline (not chlorine), and betaine can help you combat these toxins rather well. Consider taking a supplement with these nutrients.
    - Take the plastic lid off your coffee before drinking it. Or use a reusable mug; most coffee shops will be glad to fill up your mug instead.
    - Carry a glass or metal water bottle. Even if your water bottle says, "BPA free," glass or metal is always best.
    - Use wax or parchment paper to cover your food instead of plastic wrap.
    - Buy personal care products that don't contain gluten or phthalates.
    - Avoid storing food in plastic containers, and definitely don't reheat food in a plastic container. Heating plastic causes it to leach chemicals like crazy, so use glass or porcelain, please.

Heavy metals - these substances accumulate in your body because your detoxification system can't remove them very quickly. Usually, though, you can solve this problem by taking a chelating agent like activated charcoal, bentonite clay, or chlorella. If you're over 50 and you've never taken a chelating agent before, I highly recommend it. After 50 years, you probably have some heavy metals built up inside, and taking activated charcoal is a cheap and easy way to reduce your toxic exposure.

- **Lead** - found in paint and pipes before 1978.
  - o **Tips for limiting exposure:**
    - ▪ If your house is older than 1978, make sure all the lead paint and pipes have been replaced.
    - ▪ Lead is also found in some soils. If you plan to grow a garden, have your soil tested for heavy metals.
- **Mercury** - commonly found in dental fillings, fungicides, pesticides, and sizeable fatty fish (especially Tuna fish).
  - o **Tips for limiting exposure:**
    - ▪ Ask your dentist if you have mercury fillings and get them replaced as soon as possible. They could be leaching mercury vapor into your body and slowly poisoning your brain.
    - ▪ Eat small fish instead of large fish. The bigger the fish, the more mercury has accumulated over time.
- **Cadmium** - found in e-cigs, white bread, and white rice.
  - o **Tips for limiting exposure**: avoid the stuff above.
- **Arsenic -** found in brown rice (low levels)
  - o **Tips for limiting exposure:** avoid brown rice.

Mold - this sneaky toxin likes to hide out in your body, avoiding detection by doctors. But all the while, it can cause a myriad of symptoms, from food allergies to nervous system dysfunction. Unfortunately, it is very resistant to your natural detoxification strategies.
  - o **Tips for limiting exposure:**
    - ▪ Most toxic molds come from your bathroom and kitchen, so keep these areas extra clean.
    - ▪ Get air filters for your home, especially for your bedroom. You are highly susceptible to mold and aerosolized toxins while you sleep.
    - ▪ Do you feel like you have to open the windows when you return home from a vacation? If so, you may have mold overgrowth.
    - ▪ Go to normi.org or hire a home health inspector to have your home tested for mold.

Other toxins to consider:
- **Hydrocarbons/benzene**: found in the fumes coming from your gas pump, exhaust pipe, and other lighter fluids.
  - ○ **Tips for limiting exposure:**
    - ▪ Avoid lighter fluid and charcoal grilling; use wood charcoal instead.
    - ▪ When you pump gas, sit in your car with the doors closed, or stand upwind from the pump.
    - ▪ Don't leave your car in idle mode. If you plan to sit in your car for more than 10 seconds, it is best to shut it off.
- **Antibiotics**: these are especially detrimental when they are prescribed unnecessarily.
  - ○ **Tips for limiting exposure:**
    - ▪ If you are taking antibiotics, eat these foods to maintain your population of healthy gut bacteria: homemade applesauce, chicken bone broth, pomegranate juice.
    - ▪ Consider taking a safer, herbal antibiotic such as biocidin.
    - ▪ After your course of antibiotics, take a probiotic supplement for a couple more weeks so you can replenish your microbiome with good bacteria.
- **Biocides and herbicides**: these are the chemicals commonly sprayed on produce.
  - ○ **Tips for limiting exposure:**
    - ▪ Always wash your produce before eating it.
    - ▪ Eat organic when you can. Use the Environmental Working Group's "Clean Fifteen" and "Dirty Dozen" publications to help you decide which foods to buy organic.
- **UV radiation**: from airplanes, tanning salons, or excessive sun exposure. UV radiation causes DNA damage and can lead to skin cancer.
  - ○ **Tips for limiting exposure:**
    - ▪ Drink tomato or grapefruit juice one hour before you are exposed to excessive UV radiation. These fruits help protect your DNA from damage.
- **Tobacco smoke**: I wouldn't be a very good doctor if I didn't mention this one. Tobacco causes significant DNA damage, kills your stem cells, and destroys your health in more ways than I can count.
  - ○ **Tips for limiting exposure:** Don't use tobacco.

ADDENDUM #3:

MOVEMENT GAMES

Humans know how to have fun. We are the most playful and creative animals on the planet. Yet we often fail to give ourselves permission to enjoy this inborn playfulness. Once adulthood rolls around, we seem to trade in our child-like goofiness for "responsibility" and "professionalism."

But let me tell you something; your so-called responsibilities are not an excuse. Responsibilities and playfulness can exist simultaneously. In fact, adding more goofiness to your work will make you more productive, and it will help you solve problems more creatively and effectively.

So, in the following pages, I'll share with you a host of games that invite you to play like a kid again. These games are based around movement, so they let you be active without going to the gym. Also, movement games are usually social activities, so you will strengthen social bonds while you're having fun. Finally, playing games enhances learning, and adding movement to the mix will essentially hit the 'save' button on the new knowledge you gain.

When playing these games, allow yourself to be childish and goofy. You don't need to be immature; just let go of your fear of embarrassment. Have the courage to try new things, and don't worry about what people say or think. When you release your inner child, you allow yourself to feel the youthful joy that we admire in children. And when other people see how much fun you're having, I bet they'll want to join in, too.

Hang-game
Number of players: 1
Equipment needed: something to hang from (a tree branch, monkey bars, ceiling joist, etc.)

Time to harness your inner monkey. This game is simple; just see how many ways you can hang from something. Try 2 arms, 1 arm, 1 arm and 1 foot, etc. Can you hang by only 2 fingers? How about under your armpit? Be creative and explore how your body can move.

Slider push
Number of players: 1
Equipment needed: something you can slide on the ground with your foot (like a carpet slider used under furniture)

Stand on one leg with a "slide-able" object near your non-standing leg. Without putting weight on your foot, try to slide the object as far away as you can, in any direction you can think of (foreword, backward, diagonal, sideways, behind your standing leg, etc.). When you think you have gone as far as you can, mark the location and try to beat it the next time.

To make this game more challenging, try it while standing on a 2x4.

Sticky Note
Number of players: 1+   Equipment needed: sticky notes

Grab one sticky note and hold it in your hand with the sticky side facing outward. Find a spot on a wall, backboard, or archway where you can stick the sticky note. Then, try to jump as high as you can and slap the note against the wall, so it sticks. Grab a new sticky note and try again. Keep trying to get higher and higher up the wall. Maybe try running up the wall.

Over-under-game
Number of players: 1+   Equipment needed: none

Find a table, rail, bench, tree branch, whatever. Try to think of all the ways you can move over, under, or around the obstacle. With each new movement you think of, try it! How many ways can you move around the object in a fun and creative way? 10? 20? 30 ways?

If you want to play this game with a partner, you can play HORSE. One person will try to move around the object in a unique way. Then, the other person will try. If the other person cannot complete the same movement, they get an H. The game continues until one person loses 5 times and spells out all the letters in HORSE. Use any word you like to make the game shorter or longer.

Stick the Landing

Number of players: 1+   Equipment needed: none

As you walk through the forest, beach, or outdoor environment, pick a target on the ground and try to jump onto that thing. Whichever way you land, try to hold that position for 3 seconds. If you held the position, you stuck the landing!

Like the game above, you can also play HORSE with another person.

Obstacle Course

Number of players: 1+   Equipment needed: be creative!

When setting up this game, use your creative juices. Find or create obstacles to run through, climb on, crawl under, jump over, swing through, etc. Trace out the course in your mind or with string. Then, do the obstacle course! The fastest time wins. You could also award prizes for the most creative route or coolest move.

Here are some ideas for obstacles: hurdles, potato sack race, army crawl under ropes, crawl through a tube, climb to the top of a rope, climb over a trellis, jump through tires, go up and down a slide, monkey bars, swing over a "crevasse," roll down a hill, or dribble a soccer ball through a zig-zag course.

Bucket toss

Number of players: 1+
Equipment needed: multiple buckets and various balls/frisbees

Mark a line on the ground and place multiple buckets at different distances away from the line. Assign a point value for each bucket (usually, the closer buckets or bigger buckets are worth fewer points). Then, try to throw the balls or frisbees into the buckets. Each bucket you make, you get the points for that bucket. After all the balls are thrown, the player with the most points wins.

You could also arrange the buckets into a tic-tac-toe board. Then, play tic-tac-toe by trying to throw a ball into each bucket. The person who makes three buckets in the same line wins the game.

King of the line/log

Number of players: 2
Equipment needed: a surface for balancing on (e.g., A log, a 2x4 piece of lumber, a curb, or a line on the ground)

Both players will face each other while standing on a line, log, or "balance beam." They will grasp hands like they are shaking hands. Then, each player will try to force the other person to lose balance and fall off the line. The first person to fall loses.

Balance wars

Number of players: 2   Equipment needed: none

Each player will stand on one leg and stand facing each other. On the count of three, each player will try to push their opponent off-balance. The first person to touch their other leg to the ground or fall over loses.

Basketball/Soccer Mini-Golf

Number of players: 2+
Equipment needed: a basketball & hoop or a soccer ball & buckets

For basketball mini-golf, create nine holes or stations around the basketball hoop. At each station, make a rule or add an obstacle to make each shot more difficult than normal. At one station, you may have to shoot with one arm. At another station, you might have to shoot a granny shot. You get the idea.

If you make the shot on the first attempt, you get a hole in one. If you miss the shot, you must grab the rebound as quickly as possible because you have to take your next shot from wherever you get control of the ball again. If it takes you 3 shots to make it in the basket, you get a 3 for the hole. After nine holes, add up your points and see which player shot the lowest score. The lowest scorer is the winner.

For soccer mini-golf, apply the same rules, but use buckets as holes. Tip the buckets on their sides and try to kick a soccer ball into the bucket. The number of kicks it takes to get the ball in the bucket is your score for the hole. Again, the lowest score after 9 holes wins.

Hot lava tag

Number of players: 2+
Equipment needed: a playground or any playing area. Be creative!

Remember this from the playground days? The ground is lava, so you can't step foot on the ground at all. One person is the lava monster, and they try to tag the other player(s) on the playground.

A modified version of this game is *Zombie mode*. Whenever someone gets tagged, they also become "it." Eventually, there may be 5-6 lava monsters, and only one person will remain to be tagged.

Pull of the sock game

Number of players: 2+   Equipment needed: one sock per player

Each player puts on a sock, so it is halfway on their foot. On the count of three, each player does whatever they can to take off the opponent's sock. Meanwhile, they are trying to prevent their own sock from being pulled. If your sock is pulled off, you're out. The last person remaining wins.

Balloon Transfer

Number of players: 2+   Equipment needed: balloons

One person has an inflated balloon between their knees. To start the game, that player must run, hop, or shuffle the balloon over to their teammate about 10 yards away. The player cannot use their hands, and they cannot drop the balloon, or else they must start over. Once they get to their teammate, the player must transfer the balloon into the other player's legs. Again, you cannot use your hands to make this transfer. See how many times you can transfer and run the balloon across the course without dropping it.

If you want, you can make this game into a relay race. The team that transfers the balloon between every team member wins the race.

Slip n' Slide Bowling/Kickball

Number of players: 2+
Equipment needed: tarps, a hose, and a ball (or bowling pins)

For bowling, lay down a length of tarp and put some fake bowling pins on one end. Get the sprinkler out to lube up the course. Then, you act like a human bowling ball by sliding down the tarp and trying to knock down all the pins.

For kickball, lay down some tarps so that it looks like a baseball diamond. Put some bases at each corner of the diamond. Then, play standard kickball, but with the bonus of super-sliding into the base.

Outdoor Scavenger Hunt

Number of players: 2+   Equipment needed: a list of objects

Make a list of objects that can be found in your surrounding area. Have each player or team grab a bag to carry their items. Then, put a time limit on the hunt. Each person or team must try to find as many items as they can in the allotted time. The team with the most items wins.

Ninja

Number of players: 3+   Equipment needed: none

Start by holding hands and standing in a circle. Ensure that everyone is equidistant from each other, then you can release your hands.

Now, imagine your hands are your swords. The object of the game is to "chop off" the hand of another player. Every time a hand gets "chopped," the player puts their injured hand behind their back to eliminate the hand from play. If a player gets both of their hands chopped, that player is eliminated from the game completely, and the remaining players continue to play. **The most important rule of the game is that you can only move once per turn, and your movements must be one fluid motion.** For example, if I make a swipe at another player but miss entirely, I have to freeze in the position where I stopped my motion. Unless I continue to swing my arm without stopping, I have to hold the position where I first ended my movement.

On the count of three, all players must quickly assume an athletic position. Again, this needs to be done all in one motion. If you want to move your arm *and* take a step backward, you must do it simultaneously; you cannot step back and then move your arm.

Once the game has started, everyone takes turns trying to chop off another player's hand (take turns in a clockwise fashion). If you attack another player's hand on your turn, you must make one fluid swing and then freeze wherever your hand stops. And you must hit the player's hand or wrist to eliminate that hand.

While a player is trying to chop your hand, you are allowed one movement to evade the attack. Whenever you stop your fluid movement, you must freeze in the position that you stopped. All players in the attacker's striking range can also evade the strike, even if the attacker does not explicitly attack you.

Keep playing until one player is victorious.

500

Number of players: 4+   Equipment needed: a ball

Designate one player as the thrower. The rest of the players are the catchers. They stand in a group, far away from the thrower. The thrower will throw the ball high up in the air and call out a number between 0 and 500. If the thrower calls "100," the player who catches the ball gets 100 points. After each throw, the players add up their total points for the round until someone reaches 500 points. The first person to reach 500 switches positions with the thrower.

The thrower can also yell out additions to the rules, such as "300, dead or alive!" Now, the catchers don't have to catch the ball to get the points. If the ball hits the ground, it doesn't matter; the first person to get the ball in their possession will win the points.

Partner Tag/Blob Tag

Number of players: 4+   Equipment needed: none

Form teams of two players. Each team must join hands and stay joined for the entirety of the game. If they break hands, they incur a penalty, and they must remain frozen in place for 3 seconds. Every team is trying to tag each other. If a team gets tagged, they are out. Last team standing wins.

Hunger Games

Number of players: 4+
Equipment needed: fake weapons, pool noodles, balls, foam swords, garbage can lids, etc.

To start, all players will stand in a circle. At the center of the circle, all the weapons are placed in a pile called the cornucopia. Each player also has a flag or a bandana hanging from their waist.

On "Go," players can either try to get a "weapon" from the cornucopia or choose to run away. The players with weapons can try to shield or strike another player. If another player gets hit with a weapon, they can no longer use the body part that got hit. For example, if you get hit in the leg, you have to hop on one leg the rest of the game.

Players can also try to pull each other's bandanas. If a player gets their bandana pulled off their waist, they are eliminated from the game. Players cannot cover up or hold on to their bandana to prevent it from being pulled.

The last person remaining in the game is the hunger games champion.

Capture the Flag

Number of players: 4+   Equipment needed: a "flag."

Split up into two teams and divide the playing area into two equal sections. Each team will then hide their flag (or bandana or any other identifiable object) in a visible but secret location. After both teams have hidden their flag, each team will try to capture the flag and bring it across the half-line back into their territory. However, if you step foot on the other team's side, the other team can tag you. When you are tagged, you get put in "jail," which is any space that the team designates as the jail cell. To get out of jail, one of your untagged teammates can come and break you out. You both have to make it back across the line while holding hands. If you get tagged during the breakout, you both go to jail.

The first team to capture the flag and bring it back across the line without getting tagged is declared the winner.

4 Corners

Number of players: 4+   Equipment needed: none

Choose 4 corners in a room or open space and assign a color to each corner.

One person is the caller and stands in the middle of the space with their eyes closed. The caller will count to 10 and then yell out a color. If a player or players are standing in the corner that was called, they are eliminated from the game. The game continues until there is one person left standing. When there are only 2 players left, they cannot stop in the same corner together.

You can also use obstacles to make it more challenging to get to each corner. If a player doesn't make it to a corner in time, they are also eliminated.

No Holds Bar

Number of players: 7+   Equipment needed: none

Form pairs of two with one person left over. Make an imaginary circle about 20ft in diameter. Each pair will sit around the edge of the circle, with one person sitting in front of the other person. The person without a pair will stand in the middle of the circle.

The middle person will spin around with their eyes closed and point their finger straight out in front of them. When this person stops spinning, their finger will be pointing at one of the pairs sitting on the edge of the circle.

When a pair is chosen, the person sitting in front becomes the runner, and the person sitting behind becomes the holder. The goal of the runner is to try to tag the person in the middle of the circle. Meanwhile, the holder tries to do whatever he/she can to prevent the runner from tagging the center-person. The holder can hang on to the runner, pin the runner down, block the runner, etc. (Note: the person in the center does not move at all; they stay in the middle of the circle and wait to get tagged).

If the holder prevents the runner for >30 seconds, the holder wins. If the runner tags the center person, the runner wins. Then, the loser of the round will trade positions with the person in the center of the circle. Keep playing for as long as you want.

Captain's Coming/Simon Says

Number of players: 4+   Equipment needed: none

Designate one player as the captain. The rest of the players are the crew, and they are standing in front of the captain. The captain will call out different orders. Much like the game of Simon says, each order requires a specific action. If a crew member starts to do the incorrect action, they are out. During the team-based actions, one person may be left behind, and that person is out, too (or just stand off to the side for 20 seconds to make the game less competitive). The last person standing wins the prize of becoming the captain for the next round.

Here are the orders that the captain can call out and the associated actions:

To the ship: run to the captain's right
To the island: run to the captain's left
Hit the deck: lay down on your stomach as quickly as possible
Attention on deck: salute and yell, "Aye, aye captain!" – now, the players cannot move until the captain gives the order of, "At ease!" (e.g., even if the captain gives another order such as "to the ship" the crew must continue to remain at attention until told "at ease")
Row the boat: the crew must form groups of three and sing "Row, row, row your boat." Anybody who is not in a group of three is out.
The love boat: crew members grab a partner and dance. Anybody without a partner is out.
Captain's Quarters: everyone runs towards the captain.
Man-over-board: Players must find a partner as quickly as possible. One partner must lay on their stomach while the other places their foot on their partner's back and acts like they are scanning the horizon (Captain Morgan pose). People without a partner, or pairs that are too slow, are eliminated.
I need a periscope: Every player falls on their back and sticks one leg in the air. The last one to do so is eliminated.
Crow's nest: All players must find a partner. The lightest player rides on their partner's back. Those without partners or who assemble the crow's nest too slowly are eliminated.
Sick turtle: Everyone falls onto their backs and waves their hands and feet in the air.

Alternative rules: If playing in a pool, all the orders stay the same except for "hit the deck," which becomes "walk the plank." The crew members must now bob underwater.

If you want to try a more structured type of play, you could always try playing traditional sports. Joining your community recreation league is a great way to try a new sport. Or you can start your own pickup games by making a Facebook group or planning a day of the week with your friends. Social media has made it so easy to get a group of people together, so use it. And if you see a pickup game in action, don't be afraid to ask to join the fun. The worst that can happen is that someone says no.

Traditional Sports

Baseball
Basketball
Cricket
Football
Golf
Gymnastics

Hockey
Lacrosse
Martial arts
Rugby
Running
Soccer

Tennis
Volleyball
Water polo
Wrestling

Non-traditional sports

Air hockey
Archery
Ax throwing
Badminton
Bike polo
Billiards
Boxing
Broomball
Croquet
Curling
Darts
Discus throw
Dodgeball
Fencing
Field hockey
Fives
Foosball
Footgolf
Footvolley

Fricket
Frisbee golf
Futsal
Gaelic camogie
Gaelic football
Hurling
Handball
Horseshoes
Kickball
Kickboxing
Miniature golf
Netball
Paddle tennis
Paddleball
Pickleball
Pushball
Quiddich
Racquetball
Roque

Shuffleboard
Skeleton
Slamball
Snow golf
Soccer tennis
Squash
Steeplechase
Street hockey
Table tennis
Tennis polo
Tetherball
Ulama
Ultimate frisbee
Wallball
Wallyball
Whirly ball
Wiffleball
Woodball

Yard/Lawn games & Night games

Contrary to popular belief, you do not need to be drinking alcohol to play these games.

Bocce ball	Golf skeeball	Ring toss
Candyman	Gma's footsteps	Sardines
Chipper pong	KanJam	Hide-n-Seek
Cops n' Robbers	Kick the can	Spike ball
Cornhole	Kubb	Twister
Firefly	Ladder toss	Washers
Flashlight tag	Lawn bowling	Water fight
Fling a ring	Lawn darts	Yard dice
Ghost 'n Grave	Molkky/scatter	Yard pong
Giant 4 in a row	Pipe ball	
Giant Jenga	Tiki Toss	

Miscellaneous movement activities/games

In my opinion, these are different than sports because they typically don't have rules associated with them unless you are competing at a high level.

4-square	Ice climbing	Scootering
Abseiling	Ice skating	Shooting
Acro skiing	Kayak/canoeing	Skateboarding
Acro yoga	Kiteboarding	Ski/snowboarding
Aerial yoga	Kneeboarding	Slacklining
Air hockey	Laser tag	Snow biking
Mountainboarding	Logrolling	Stilts
Backpacking	Long-boarding	Surf/bodyboarding
Balance boarding	Luge	Trampolining
Bouldering	Miniature golf	Trapeze
Bull riding	Mountain biking	Tree climbing
Canyoneering	Paddle boarding	Unicycling
Crosscountry skiing	Paintballing	Wakeboarding
Cycling	Parkour	Water-skiing
Dancing	Rock climbing	Whitewater rafting
Fishing	Rollerblading	Wind/Kitesurfing
Geocaching	Rope climbing	Zorbing
Grass skiing	Rowing	
Hunting	Sandboarding	

Video games

Outdoor games are ideal, but certain video games will still get you moving, too. Xbox Kinect and the Wii are a couple of examples, but make sure that the games you buy are movement-based.

ADDENDUM #4:

MOBILITY CHECK-UP

Movement is our expression of life. It allows us the freedom to explore the world, play with our kids, and dance with our loved ones. Unfortunately, as we age, many of us lose our ability to enjoy these activities. At one point, you may have made an excuse that "I just can't move like that anymore." But instead of doing anything about it, we chalk it up to the "natural" aging process.

Well, let me tell you; there is nothing natural about something like relying on a walker just to get to the bathroom. And if you keep making excuses for your lack of mobility, that may be where you are headed. Immobility may be common in our society, but it's not natural. Your body is a movement machine, and it was built to last. In fact, moving your body is usually what keeps you alive for so long. To rephrase a quote by Mr. Andy Dufresne, "you either get busy moving, or you get busy dying."

But just because you've lost some mobility doesn't mean you're headed for an early grave. You can get your mobility back, and I'm here to help you. No matter your age, I believe you can turn your health around and get back to doing any activity you want.

The first step to improving your mobility is to keep track of it. In this mobility check-up, you will perform 12 foundational movements to assess your mobility and movement quality. These are called 'foundational movements' because they are stripped-down versions of almost any activity that you can imagine. Whether you want to play competitive sports, garden, or simply get out of a chair, the basic movements in this check-up will lay the groundwork. By stripping down your daily activities into foundational movements, you can see if you have any limitations. These limitations may be the reason why you can't do the tasks you once enjoyed. Or, your limitations may be impeding your athletic performance and increasing your risk of injury, thus predisposing you to future immobility.

If you discover that you cannot do one or more of the activities in this check-up, don't worry. The inability to perform a movement does not mean you are broken or dysfunctional; it just means that you haven't exposed yourself to those movements in a while. Movement is a nutrient, and you may be a little malnourished, but you're not yet starving.

With that said, your movement limitation should not be taken lightly. If you can't even do the basic movements in this check-up, then what will it look like when you do more complex tasks in your daily life? Most likely, it won't look good. Your body will compensate with inefficient body mechanics that put abnormal stresses on different tissues of your body. If you keep that up, you'll probably end up getting injured, and the pain will cause more compensations, more dysfunctions, and more injuries, thus starting the cycle all over again.

Even minor injuries can build on each other until you slowly lose the mobility that you once had. Without realizing what is happening, you'll stop doing the activities you used to enjoy. Then, your mobility will get worse because you won't be moving as much throughout the day. Eventually, you could end up stuck in that bed in the nursing home because you can't even walk on your own anymore.

Sorry to be so dramatic, but this stuff is important. Without mobility, you lose your independence, your quality of life, and your reason for living. How do you expect to live a full and youthful life if you can't walk on your own two feet?

Thankfully, you have plenty of time to get your mobility back. And for most people, the solution to a movement problem is the same; move more often! For some, that means spending more time doing specific movements. For others, it means they just need to get off the couch and do something, anything. In my experience, it's both. The type of person who achieves Lifelong Youth is active and moving for most of their day. And when movement limitations come up, they spend a little extra time with targeted exercises that improve their mobility.

As you begin to work on your movement limitations, you may find that you can perform activities you used to enjoy but had to give up. You may find that your bodily aches and pains go away. One thing is for sure, improving your mobility skills will help you live life to the fullest, free to do any activity that you set your mind to, and with the youthful exuberance of your 20-year-old self. Okay, maybe I'm acting dramatic again, but you get the point.

Note:
The mobility check-up is on video! You can follow along by going to lifelongyouthbook.com/resources, where you can also print out the full mobility check-up along with the score sheets.

Before You Begin

The movements in this mobility check-up progress from easiest to hardest. As you seek to improve your movement capacity, it is best to start your journey from the ground up. If you find that you cannot do a task at the beginning of this workbook, try to improve your mobility in that area first. Then, you can progress to more challenging activities. In other words, you need to crawl before you can walk and walk before you can run.

If you notice a difference between your right and left sides during a movement, those discrepancies take priority. For instance, let's say you fail the squat test. Then on the lunge test, you pass on the right leg but fail on the left leg. You pass all remaining screens.
Even though the squat test shows up earlier than the lunge, the movement asymmetry is more important than a failed movement. Therefore, you should work on your lunge discrepancy first.
Besides, improving a movement asymmetry often ends up improving other movements simultaneously. So, by fixing your lunge, your squat test might improve, too.

To summarize, when you have more than one failed movement, start with the asymmetrical movements first. Then, work on the movements at the beginning of this workbook before you progress to the more challenging movements. Take it one step at a time and work from the ground up. Skipping to the most challenging task will often result in compensations, which lead to injuries down the road. You don't want to take one leap forward, get injured, and fall eight steps behind. Take your time to progress appropriately. If you need to, call upon a movement specialist in your area to help determine the appropriate progression for you.

Required Tools

- A doorway (3' wide)
- A dowel or broomstick (about 4' long)
- A roll of tape or string
- A tape measurer
- A pen, pencil, or sharpie (for writing on the tape/string)
- A scoresheet (on the following page)

References and Inspirations

The ideas in this mobility check-up are not my own; they are a compilation of ideas from much smarter people than me. Below is a brief list of the people who inspired this mobility check-up and are responsible for developing the movement screens that I describe.

- Gray Cook and Lee Burton - from Functional Movement Systems. Gray Cook is the author of 'Movement' [352] and 'Athletic Body and Balance.' [353] These two individuals get most of the credit for designing the movement screens in this workbook.
- Craig Liebenson - from First Principles of Movement and author of 'The Functional Training Handbook.' [354]
- Erwan LeCorre - from MoveNat and author of 'The Practice of Natural Movement.' [355]
- Kelly Starrett - from 'The Ready State' and author of 'Becoming a Supple Leopard.' [356]
- Rafe Kelley - from EvolveMovePlay

Safety Note:

This 'Mobility Check-up' is not a medical evaluation. If you are recovering from an injury or currently have pain, the mobility check-up is NOT for you; you need a complete musculoskeletal evaluation to identify and explain your problem. If you do not have pain or a preexisting problem but experience pain during the mobility check-up, you would also benefit from a complete musculoskeletal evaluation. If you plan to initiate a new training program or start a new activity, try to pass all the movements in this mobility check-up first. Training on top of immobility or movement discrepancies can lead to future injury or dysfunction.

Scoring Sheet

The scoring system is simple. If you complete the movement and meet all the criteria, you get a pass. If you cannot complete the movement within the criteria provided, you receive a *fail* for the movement. If you have pain during any activity, I recommend that you have a medical professional perform a thorough evaluation. A feeling of stretch is defined as discomfort, whereas any other sensation is considered pain.

Test	Side	Pass	Fail	Comments
Breathing	-			
Ground Get Up	-			
Active SLR	L			
	R			
Toe Touch	-			
Wall Angel	-			
Deep Squat	-			
Hurdle Step	L			
	R			
In-line Lunge	L			
	R			
Standing/Seated Rotation	L			
	R			
Trunk Stability Push-Up	-			
Rotary Stability	L			
	R			

		Average of 3 attempts in each direction		Comments
Y-Balance Test	L	Direction 1 =	cm	
		Direction 2 =	cm	
		Direction 3 =	cm	
	R	Direction 1 =	cm	
		Direction 2 =	cm	
		Direction 3 =	cm	

Breathing

Breathing doesn't sound like much of a mobility exercise, but it underpins every movement you perform. If you are not breathing efficiently, your muscles, brain, nerves, and organs may not get the oxygen they need to do their jobs. Plus, improper breathing can make some muscles in your body work harder than they need to, which can create painful problems in your back and neck as well as your shoulders and hips.

Performing the "movement":

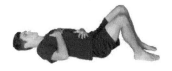

- Lie on your back with your legs bent and feet flat on the floor.
- Put one hand on the top of your chest and the other hand over your belly button.
- Breathe normally, not too big, or too shallow, just a relaxed, full breath.
- Did you notice which hand moved the most? Was it your chest hand or your belly hand?
- Take a couple more breaths and pay attention to your hands. Which hand moves first? Which hand moves the most?

Scoring:

- Pass
  - Your belly hand moved first and most, and your chest hand moved very slightly (if at all).

Proper breathing means primarily using your diaphragm so that your belly pushes outward, and your lower ribcage expands sideways. Improper breathing is when your chest and shoulders rise with each breath. Your chest should only be rising at the deepest part of your breath, and your belly should move during most of the breath.

- Fail
  - Your chest hand moved first and most, and your belly hand hardly moved.

If you have pain during this assessment, I recommend that you have a medical professional perform a thorough evaluation.

As Gray Cook says, if you can't breathe during a movement, you don't "own the movement." So, for the rest of the movements in this check-up, always remember to take full breaths. You should be able to breathe at about 80-90% of your maximum capacity, primarily through your belly. If you can't perform the movement and breathe simultaneously, you are likely compensating with inefficient body mechanics. In short, if you can't breathe deeply during the movement, you haven't mastered it yet.

Ground Get Up

Getting off the ground is an act of strength, stability, and balance. It is also a predictor of longevity. Those who can get up off the ground without using their hands end up living longer than their "less athletic" peers.[357] It may seem like a trivial test, but it speaks volumes for those of us on a mission to achieve Lifelong Youth.

Performing the movement:
- Sit on the ground.
- Without using your hands, try to stand up from the ground.
- If you can't get up, try assisting with one arm.
- You have up to three chances to complete the test.

Scoring:
- Pass
  - You can get up off the ground without using your arms.
- Tentative pass
  - You need to use one arm to help get up. You still pass this screen, but I believe you can do it no-handed if you work at it.
- Fail
  - You cannot get off the ground without needing both arms to assist you.
  - You cannot breathe to 80% capacity while performing the movement.

If you have pain during this assessment, I recommend that you have a medical professional perform a thorough evaluation.

Active Straight-Leg Raise (SLR)

You've probably never done this movement in your daily life. But the ability to bring your leg beyond 70 degrees of hip flexion will help you be more efficient when walking, running, and playing sports.

Performing the movement:

- Lie on your back with your body perpendicular to the doorway. Your legs should be flat, and the middle of your outside thigh should be touching the doorframe.
- Keep your arms at your sides, palms up, head flat on the floor, and your feet together with toes pointing up.
- Now, while keeping your knee straight, lift the leg that is touching the door frame. Lift that leg as far as you can while keeping the knee extended. Your opposite leg should remain flat on the floor and not bend or move at all.
- Shift to the opposite doorframe and perform the same movement with the other leg.
- You have up to three chances to complete the test.

Scoring: the leg that is being lifted in the air is the side of scoring

- Pass
    - You can lift your leg past the door jamb without moving any other body part. Use the outside of your ankle as a measuring device. If the knobby bone on the outside of the ankle clears the door jam, you pass.

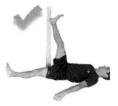

- Fail
    - The outside of your ankle cannot clear the door jam.
    - You cannot clear the door jamb without moving your other body parts. For example, your arms do not remain palm up, you lift your head off the ground, or your opposite knee bends during the movement.

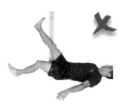

    - You may feel your low back arching a lot during this movement. Or you might feel your butt pushing hard into the ground. This means you are using your hip flexors without stabilizing your core, and this also receives a failing score.
    - You cannot breathe to 80% capacity while performing the movement.

If you have pain during this assessment, I recommend that you have a medical professional perform a thorough evaluation.

Toe Touch

Such a simple task, and yet many people cannot touch their toes. Touching your toes is one of the most practical movement skills; you perform it several times per day when grabbing items off the ground, putting on your socks, and tying your shoes. Also, this movement resembles the traditional deadlift, which is one of the most fundamental lifting skills. Therefore, getting this movement right is an essential step in your mobility journey.

Performing the movement:

- Stand (no shoes) with your feet and knees together.
- Place your hands on the front of your thighs.
- While keeping your knees extended, slide your hands as far down your legs as possible and attempt to touch your toes.
- You have up to three chances to complete the test.

Scoring:

- Pass
  - You can touch your toes while keeping your knees straight.
- Fail

  - You cannot touch your toes.
  - Your knees bend before touching your toes.
  - You cannot breathe to 80% capacity while performing the movement.

If you have pain during this assessment, I recommend that you have a medical professional perform a thorough evaluation.

Wall angel

This movement combines mobility skills in the shoulder, shoulder blade, and mid-back (thoracic spine). Thoracic and shoulder mobility are intimately connected, so if you have shoulder problems, your thoracic spine may be the source. Also, the shoulder blade is a unique connection point between the thoracic spine and the shoulder. Proper shoulder motion relies entirely on the shoulder blade, and yet dysfunctions in the shoulder blade are common, especially in sedentary people who slouch all day. Performing this wall angel can help you see if all those structures are working together or not.

Performing the movement:

- Stand with your back flat against a wall. Tilt your pelvis so the small of your back is flat. Do not stick your belly out.
- Move your feet about 1-2 feet away from the wall and shoulder-width apart.
- Your buttocks and the back of your head should be against the wall. Tuck your chin so you maintain a horizontal gaze.
- Make a "field goal" sign with your arms by making a "T" and then bending your elbows to 90 degrees.
- Your elbows and all five fingers should be touching the wall.
- Now, try to flatten your wrist while keeping your fingers and elbows against the wall.
- You have up to three chances to complete the test.

Scoring:

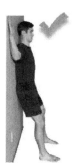

- Pass
  - You can touch your wrists to the wall while keeping the other contact points against the wall: fingers, elbows, head, buttocks, and low back.
  - You do not need to arch your back to accomplish the movement.
- Fail
  - You are unable to touch your wrists to the wall.
  - You cannot maintain the other contact points while attempting to touch your wrists to the wall.
  - You cannot breathe to 80% capacity while performing the movement.

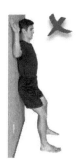

If you have pain during this assessment, I recommend that you have a medical professional perform a thorough evaluation.

Deep Squat

The squat test is one of the most important tests in the mobility check-up. We need to squat for many daily activities like getting out of a chair, lifting objects, and assuming the "athletic position" in sports.

Not everyone will be able to squat the same depth or in the same way, but there are certain squatting standards that everyone should meet. If you want to perform basic daily activities safely and efficiently, you ought to pass the squat assessment.

Performing the movement:

- Place a 12-inch strip of tape in the doorway, about one shoe-length away from the door frame.
- Now, stand (no shoes) with your feet shoulder-width apart and both big toes touching the strip of tape. You should be facing the door frame closest to you. Half of your body should be on each side of the door.
- Hold a dowel overhead with both hands. Your hands should be a little wider than shoulder-width apart.
    If you hit the top of the door with the dowel, finish extending your elbows as you descend into the squat position.
- Once you are in the proper position, descend slowly into a full squat position as deep as you can go. As you descend, your heels should be flat, and your feet should not slide or move outward.
- The dowel should remain overhead during the squat. Do not touch the doorframe with the dowel or any part of your body.
- You have up to three chances to complete the test.

Scoring:

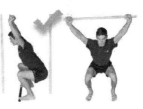

- Pass
    o Heels remain on the floor, and your feet do not slide or rotate.
    o The dowel remains maximally pressed overhead and does not touch the wall.
    o Your hips can fall below your knees.
    o Your knees stay aligned over the feet.
- Fail
    o You cannot achieve the elements above.
    o You cannot breathe to 80% capacity while performing the movement.

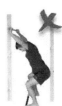

If you have pain during this assessment, I recommend that you have a medical professional perform a thorough evaluation.

Hurdle Step

This basic movement is foundational for activities such as climbing stairs, hiking, stepping onto a stool, and maintaining balance during any one-legged activity. This screen also tests for proper mobility, stability, posture, and coordination between the lower body and core.

Performing the movement:

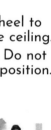

- Place a strip of tape across a doorway to create a hurdle. Align the hurdle's height with the bump on your upper shin, just below the kneecap (aka *tibial tuberosity*).
- Position a dowel across your shoulders (not your neck).
- Stand (no shoes) in the doorway, facing the tape. Place your feet together. Align the tops of your toes to be directly under the tape. In this position, the dowel should be just behind the door.
- Stand with a tall spine.
- Now, slowly step one foot over the tape and touch your heel to the floor on the other side. Keep your toes pointed at the ceiling.
- On the other side of the tape, tap your heel to the floor. Do not put weight on your stepping foot. Return to the starting position.
- Perform the same movement on the other side.
- You have up to three chances to complete the test.

Scoring: the leg you stand on is the side of scoring

- Pass
  - Your hips, knees, and ankles remain forward.
  - The dowel and hurdle remain parallel. In other words, the dowel cannot dip to the left or the right. There should be little to no movement above the waist. Balance is maintained.
  - The dowel does not touch the wall (this would happen if you leaned forward).
- Fail
  - You cannot achieve the elements above, or you lose balance.
  - You cannot clear the tape and touch your heel to the other side.
  - You cannot breathe to 80% capacity while performing the movement.
- Be critical of yourself. If you have to contort your body to get over the tape, then you have identified a problem to be corrected.

If you have pain during this assessment, I recommend that you have a medical professional perform a thorough evaluation.

In-line lunge

The lunge is a useful movement to keep your body safe. You perform a modified lunge when you catch yourself from falling and when you change directions quickly. The lunge movement is also useful for lifting objects off the ground, throwing, tying your shoes, and performing ground activities like gardening or cleaning.

Performing the movement:

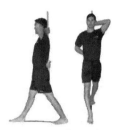

- Cut a strip of tape that is the length of your foot up to your kneecap. Place the tape on the floor.
- Stand (no shoes) on the tape in a split stance position. The toes of your back leg should just barely be touching the back of the tape. The heel of your front leg should touch the front edge of the tape.
- Grab a dowel and place it behind your back, so it touches the back of your head, your upper back, and your tailbone.
- Grab the top of the dowel with the hand that is opposite to your front foot (if your right leg is forward, grab the top of the dowel with your left hand). This hand should be holding the dowel just behind the curve of your neck.
- With your other hand, grab the bottom of the dowel. This hand should be holding the dowel just behind the curve of your low back.
- Now perform a lunge movement. Lower your back knee to the ground so that you just barely touch the tape with your knee. Then return to the starting position while maintaining a tall spine.
- Perform the same movement with the other leg forward. Remember to switch your hands on the dowel, too.
- You have up to three chances to complete the test.

Scoring: the front leg identifies the side you are scoring

- Pass

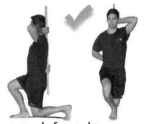

  o The heel of your front foot should remain flat on the floor.
  o Your toes remain straight. Your feet do not slide or move off the tape during the movement.
  o The dowel remains in contact with your head, upper back, and tailbone.
  o The dowel remains upright and does not tip left, right, or forward. In other words, you have little to no upper body motion. You also do not lose grip of the dowel.

- Fail
    - The elements above cannot be achieved.
    - You fall over, lose balance, or move your feet too much.
    - You cannot breathe to 80% capacity while performing the movement.

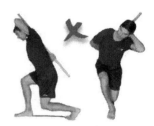

If you have pain during this assessment, I recommend that you have a medical professional perform a thorough evaluation.

Standing and Seated Rotation

Everyone's gotta turn. From checking your blind spot to swinging a golf club, rotating from the standing or seated position is an essential function. Being able to rotate in a controlled manner is also safer for your back and neck. And with more control over your back, you gain more power and control in your extremities. Therefore, rotational control means full-body control.

Performing the movement:

- Sit in the middle of the doorway, with your legs crossed, facing the doorframe. Sit upright with a tall spine.
- Hold a dowel on your chest so that it touches both collarbones and the front of both shoulders. Cross your arms to hold the dowel.
- With a tall spine, rotate to each side. Attempt to touch the dowel to the door frame in front of you. Do not lean forward or bend your spine sideways.
- Do not try to force it. You should be able to complete this movement without winding up or giving a final push.
- For the standing rotation, start with your feet together, standing in the middle of the door, facing the door frame. Without moving your feet, rotate your shoulders to each side as far as you can. Keep a tall spine, and don't try to force the movement.
- You have up to three chances to complete the test.

Scoring: the side that you rotate toward is the side of scoring

- Pass
  - You can rotate far enough so your shoulder (or dowel) can reach beyond the door frame (or touches the door frame).
  - Your spine remains tall and upright, without bending to the side or backward. The dowel remains level and in contact with your chest.
  - You can complete the movement in one fluid motion without having to force it.
- Fail
  - You cannot reach your shoulder past the door frame while maintaining the elements listed above. If sitting, you cannot touch the dowel to the doorframe in front of you.
  - You cannot breathe to 80% capacity while performing the movement.

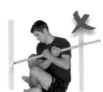

If you have pain during this assessment, I recommend that you have a medical professional perform a thorough evaluation.

Trunk stability push-up

This test is used to assess core control. Good control over your trunk and core translates into power, strength, and coordination in your arms and legs. Since virtually every human activity requires arms and legs, core control is essential for optimal performance and injury prevention.

Performing the movement:

- Lie face down with arms extended overhead at shoulder-width apart.
- Pull your thumbs down in line with your forehead (for men) or chin (for women).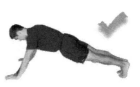
- Bring your legs together and rest on your toes, like you are about to do a push-up.
- Extend your knees and lift your elbows slightly off the ground.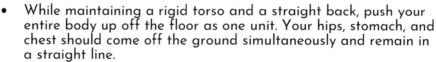
- While maintaining a rigid torso and a straight back, push your entire body up off the floor as one unit. Your hips, stomach, and chest should come off the ground simultaneously and remain in a straight line.
- You have up to three chances to complete the test.

Scoring:

- Pass
  - You can push up while maintaining a rigid spine and torso. Your chest, stomach, and hips come off the ground simultaneously.
  - Your body does not sway, tilt, or bend to one side during the movement
- Fail
  - You cannot perform a push-up while maintaining a rigid torso.
  - Your chest, stomach, and hips lift off the ground at different times. Or your body bends, tilts, and sways while attempting the push-up.
  - You cannot breathe to 80% capacity while performing the movement.

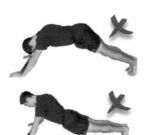

If you have pain during this assessment, I recommend that you have a medical professional perform a thorough evaluation.

Rotary stability

Similar to the trunk stability push-up, rotary stability assesses for core control. This time, though, you will combine upper and lower body movements. Your daily activities often rely on your upper and lower limbs working simultaneously, and your core should stabilize during those activities. If your core is not stable, you may be placing improper loads on your body and increasing your risk for injury. This assessment will help you determine if your core stability is keeping you safe or lying down on the job.

Performing the movement:

- Put a strip of tape or a dowel on the floor
- Get on your hands and knees and align your body so that the line splits your body in half, lengthwise.
- Place your hands directly under your shoulders and your knees directly under your hips. Your thumbs, knees, and toes must contact the sides of the line/dowel.
- Pull your toes toward your shins, so you are resting on your toes. Keep a neutral neck, so you are looking at the ground.
- Now, in one fluid motion, reach your right hand forward and your left leg backward at the same time (your arm and leg should form a straight line at the end of the movement). Act like you are pushing a box away from you in both directions.
- Without touching the ground, bring your arm and leg back together and touch your right elbow to your left knee.
- Your elbow and knee should be touching directly over the line beneath you.
- Reach with your arm and leg one more time. Return to start.
- Perform the same motion on the other side (left arm & right leg).
- You have up to three chances to complete the test

Scoring: the side of the moving leg is the side of scoring

- Pass
  - You can touch your elbow and knee together while staying directly over the line/dowel.
- Fail
  - You are unable to touch your elbow to your knee, or you lose balance during the movement.
  - You cannot breathe to 80% capacity while performing the movement.

If you have pain during this assessment, I recommend that you have a medical professional perform a thorough evaluation.

Y-balance

The Y-balance test is by far the most challenging test in the mobility check-up. It is a useful tool for measuring your risk of injury, especially if you like to play high-impact sports. The test combines many different elements of movement that you are guaranteed to need in your daily life. These components include postural control, range of motion, and balance.

Note: you will need a partner, a tape measurer, tape/string, and a pen/pencil.

Performing the movement:

• Place three, 4 feet long strips of tape/string on the ground to form a Y. The fork on the Y should make a 90-degree angle.

• Stand (no shoes) with the edge of your heel on the intersection of tape. Face the trunk/base of the Y.

• While standing on one leg, reach with your other leg as far as you can over the tape.

• DO NOT put any weight on your reaching leg. You may only touch the tape lightly with your toes. If you lose balance or put weight on your reaching leg, restart the movement.

• To get the hang of the movement, you can practice reaching 1-2 times in each direction. Once you start the test, you have 3 attempts to reach as far as you can in every direction.

• Now, start the movement. Place your hands on your hips and reach with one leg in every direction, starting with the forward reach. You can bend your knee as far as you need to, but you cannot lift your heel off the ground.

• When you have reached as far as you can, have your partner put a mark on the tape.

• Return to the starting position after each reach attempt. After 3 attempts, perform the reach in the next direction.

• Measure your distances (in cm). For each direction, take the average of your 3 attempts and record the score in your scoresheet. The leg you were standing on is the side of scoring.

• Switch legs and repeat the test. Again, calculate the average distance achieved in each direction.

Scoring: the standing leg is the side of scoring

- Pass
  - When comparing your right and left leg, the difference between your average scores should be within certain parameters.
  - **Forward reach**: your right and left leg averages are within **4 cm.**
  - **Backward reaches** (in either direction): your right and left leg averages are within **6 cm.**
  - For example, in the reaching forward direction, you scored 50cm while standing on the right leg and 47cm when standing on the left leg. These measurements are within 4 cm, so you pass.
- Fail
  - You have an asymmetry of greater than **4 cm** when reaching forward or greater than **6cm** when reaching backward (in either direction).
  - You cannot breathe to 80% capacity while performing the movement.

If you have pain during this assessment, I recommend that you have a medical professional perform a thorough evaluation.

Mobility Check-up FAQ's

How often should I do the mobility check-up?
I recommend once a month. After a couple of runs through the full mobility check-up, it should only take you about 15 minutes to perform the whole thing. I also recommend keeping a record of your scores and measurements so you can track your progress.

How long will it take to correct a failed mobility exercise?
Many movement patterns will change quickly; others will change very little. Your diligence, lifestyle habits, genetics, and other biopsychosocial factors will dictate how quickly your mobility will improve. Still, you can expect most movement patterns to improve within two months of corrective exercise work.

If I failed a movement, what should I do to improve my score?
The easy answer to this question is "corrective exercises." The long answer would require an entire book and would still be inadequate for your unique scenario. The truth is, to improve your mobility, you'll need a personalized plan that fits with your lifestyle and goals. If you want help creating a personalized plan, look for a chiropractor, physical therapist, coach, or personal trainer in your area.

For now, you can use these guidelines to help improve your mobility:

- If you fail a movement, do that movement more often in your daily life. You don't need to do it exactly how it's described in this mobility checkup; just do something similar. For example, when you are out on your daily walk, do a few lunges now and then. When you are brushing your teeth, stand on one leg and do a couple of hurdle steps. The key is to play around with these movements in your daily life, so you expose your body to all of its capabilities. As you continue to do more unique movements, your body will realize that you need more mobility in your daily life, and your body will adapt to make you more mobile. If you don't move very often, your body will take your mobility back. What's the point of keeping your body mobile if you are never going to need it?

- For those of you who like more direction, there are plenty of videos on the internet that will guide you through mobility exercises for different body parts. Most of these will do just fine for improving your mobility, but they will not work in isolation. You have to use your newfound mobility in your daily life if you want it to stick. Doing 10 minutes of mobility work will not make up for the 10 hours you spent sitting in a chair or couch.

- Use these resources to find specific corrective exercises for your movement discrepancy: functionalmovement.com/exercises; mytpi.com/exercises

If I have a movement discrepancy, do I have to stop my activities until I can perform that movement?

Sorry, but my answer is, "it depends." If your daily activities are low to moderate intensity, your movement discrepancies may not be an issue. However, suppose you are adding a lot of weight or load onto a movement (like lifting weights, moving heavy boxes, running longer distances, etc.). In that case, you should try to resolve your movement discrepancy before you try to progress to more intense activity. As Gray Cook puts it, you need to move well, first, then you can move often. By training on top of a dysfunctional or painful movement, you set yourself up for injury or disability because your body is probably compensating with a sub-optimal movement. This will make your muscles and joints work too hard or in incorrect ways. If you want more help, look for a chiropractor, physical therapist, coach, or personal trainer to help you on your journey.

My mobility is not improving; what should I do differently?

If your progress feels stalled, or if you want quicker results, talk to a movement specialist. Chiropractors, physical therapists, coaches, and personal trainers are useful because they can help find limitations that prevent or impede your movement progress and then develop a program to overcome those obstacles. Make sure you choose the right provider, though. Look for someone who emphasizes movement in their marketing. And if you are moving a lot during the assessment and examination process, you are probably in the right place.

Why can't I do movement 'xyz' in the mobility check-up?

Remember, the mobility check-up is not a medical evaluation; you need a complete musculoskeletal exam to identify and explain your problem. Since you are a unique person with a unique history, I cannot say why you have developed this particular movement discrepancy. However, I can say that movement patterns often develop from your daily habits, activities, and previous injuries. The more you perform a habit or activity, you engrave that movement pattern deeper into your brain. Contrarily, a lack of activity allows some movement patterns to deteriorate. Also, your past injuries may not be fully rehabilitated, and thus your brain is still protecting your "injured" area by putting limitations on its mobility or stability.

How is it possible that I can perform complex activities like playing sports or lifting really heavy objects, but I can't do these simple bodyweight movements?

Many people can perform a wide range of activities, yet they cannot execute the movements in the mobility check-up. Those who score poorly on the screens are using compensatory movement patterns during their regular activities. If these compensations continue, sub-optimal movement patterns are reinforced, leading to poor biomechanics and possibly future injury.

Also, regarding weight-training, most weightlifting/exercise programs are targeted at specific muscles and muscle groups. This exercise style is called *isolation training*, and even though it is useful for building muscle, those muscles are kind of stupid. They are good at lifting weights in a specific way, but they are not good at performing functional movements. This may be why you see top-level weightlifters who can't do a simple task like putting their hand on their spine. A recent shift in weightlifting is now prioritizing functional training for physical performance rather than muscle gains. Physical performance is more focused on movement development, which is not the same as muscular development. Physical performance is about muscles working together rather than isolating individual muscles. If you train functional movements for physical performance, you will train your body to be highly mobile and agile, and your muscles will develop appropriately. Those muscles will look just as good without a shirt on, too.

Why do all these movements keep telling me to have a straight spine? Isn't my spine supposed to bend and move?

Yes, your spine is supposed to bend and move. With just your bodyweight, your spine should be flexible enough to bend, twist, and move around freely so it can adapt to many different situations. However, when you start doing more intense, complex activities (like shoveling dirt, playing sports, or carrying heavy objects), having a sturdy spine will protect you from injury, improve your performance, and waste less energy.

Most forceful movements that produce power, speed, agility, and quickness require the extremities (the arms and legs) to move freely while the spine is maintained in a tall, erect posture. In other words, your spine should be stable enough to support the body while your extremities do the work of transferring power. Therefore, training for mobility and stability means practicing the mechanics of having a tall, erect spine. That way, when you come across a complex task, your brain remembers a safe and efficient movement pattern rather than relying on a compensatory and potentially dangerous movement pattern.

What if I have pain during a movement?

If you have pain with any of the movements in this mobility check-up, without a doubt, you should schedule an appointment with a specialist. Chiropractors and physical therapists are considered the first line of defense for pain associated with movement. Both practitioners offer exceptionally safe yet effective treatments that can help you get back to the activities you enjoy.

The End!

Resources/Acknowledgements

If you'd like to dive deeper into the wonderful world of health and longevity, consider these resources. I owe a lot of thanks to the minds that decided to share these ideas with the world.

Books

- 7 Habits of Highly Effective People - Stephen Covey
- Atomic Habits - James Clear
- The Auto-immune Fix - Tom O'Bryan, DC
- Becoming a Supple Leopard - Kelly Starrett
- The Big Fat Surprise - Nina Teicholz
- The Blue Zones Series - Dan Buettner
- Brain Maker - David Perlmutter
- The Disease Delusion - Jeffrey Bland
- The Doctor's Farmacy Podcast - Mark Hyman
- Eat More, Weigh Less - Dean Ornish
- Eat to Beat Disease - William Li
- Genius Foods - Max Lugavere
- Getting Things Done - David Allen
- Good Calories, Bad Calories - Gary Taubes
- Grain Brain - David Perlmutter
- Lifespan - David Sinclair
- The Plant Paradox - Steven Gundry
- The Longevity Paradox - Steven Gundry
- Movement - Gray Cook
- The Omnivore's Dilemma - Michael Pollan
- Playing with Movement - Todd Hargrove
- The Power of Habit - Charles Duhigg
- The Practice of Natural Movement - Erwan Le Corre
- Thrive - Dan Buettner
- Undo it - Dean Ornish
- The Wahls Protocol - Terry Wahls
- Wheat Belly - William Davis
- Why Zebras Don't Get Ulcers - Robert Sapolsky
- You Can Fix Your Brain - Tom O'Bryan, DC

Online

- Americangrassfed.org
- Bluezones.com
- Eatwild.com
- Firsthandfoods.org
- Functionalmovement.com/exercises
- https://www.ewg.org/foodnews/clean-fifteen.php
- https://www.ewg.org/foodnews/dirty-dozen.php;
- https://www.ewg.org/foodnews/summary.php
- Ifm.org
- Localharvest.com
- Lpi.oregonstate.edu
- Mytpi.com/exercises
- Movenat.com
- Pubmed.gov
- theDr.com/readyquiz
- Thereadystate.com
- Thrivemarket.com

Follow Us!

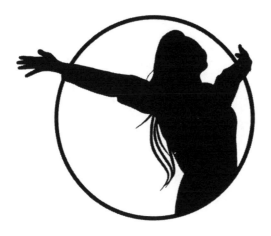

Web: lifelongyouthbook.com

facebook.com/LifelongYouth

instagram.com/mylifelongyouth/

Reference List

[1] FastStats - Life Expectancy. Centers for Disease Control and Prevention. https://www.cdc.gov/nchs/fastats/life-expectancy.htm. Published March 17, 2017. Accessed March 29, 2020.

[2] Roser M, Ortiz-Ospina E, Ritchie H. Life Expectancy. Our World in Data. https://ourworldindata.org/life-expectancy. Published May 23, 2013. Accessed March 29, 2020.

[3] Ludwig DS. Childhood Obesity – The Shape of Things to Come. *New England Journal of Medicine*. 2007;357(23):2325-2327. doi:10.1056/nejmp0706538.

[4] Determinants of Health Visualized. Visualized. https://www.goinvo.com/vision/determinants-of-health/. Accessed March 29, 2020.

[5] WHO, NCHHSTP, Healthy People, Kaiser Family, NEJM, Health Affairs, Institute of Medicine, & New South Wales Department of Health

[6] 2018 Global Nutrition Report reveals malnutrition is unacceptably high and affects every country in the world, but there is also an unprecedented opportunity to end it. UNICEF. https://www.unicef.org/press-releases/2018-global-nutrition-report-reveals-malnutrition-unacceptably-high-and-affects. Accessed March 29, 2020.

[7] Panula J, Pihlajamäki H, Mattila VM, et al. Mortality and cause of death in hip fracture patients aged 65 or older: a population-based study. *BMC Musculoskelet Disord*. 2011;12:105. Published 2011 May 20. doi:10.1186/1471-2474-12-105

[8] Li WW. *Eat to Beat Disease: the New Science of How the Body Can Heal Itself*. New York: Grand Central Publishing; 2019.

[9] Young VB. The role of the microbiome in human health and disease: an introduction for clinicians. *BMJ*. 2017;356:j831. Published 2017 Mar 15. doi:10.1136/bmj.j831

[10] Singer-Englar T, Barlow G, Mathur R. Obesity, diabetes, and the gut microbiome: an updated review. *Expert Rev Gastroenterol Hepatol*. 2019;13(1):3-15. doi:10.1080/17474124.2019.1543023

[11] Young VB. The role of the microbiome in human health and disease: an introduction for clinicians. *BMJ*. 2017;356:j831. Published 2017 Mar 15. doi:10.1136/bmj.j831

[12] Sajib S, Zahra FT, Lionakis MS, German NA, Mikelis CM. Mechanisms of angiogenesis in microbe-regulated inflammatory and neoplastic conditions. *Angiogenesis*. 2018;21(1):1-14. doi:10.1007/s10456-017-9583-4

[13] Zimmermann M, Zimmermann-Kogadeeva M, Wegmann R, Goodman AL. Mapping human microbiome drug metabolism by gut bacteria and their genes. *Nature*. 2019;570(7762):462-467. doi:10.1038/s41586-019-1291-3

[14] Obrenovich MEM. Leaky Gut, Leaky Brain?. *Microorganisms*. 2018;6(4):107. Published 2018 Oct 18. doi:10.3390/microorganisms6040107

[15] Plaza-Diaz J, Gomez-Llorente C, Fontana L, Gil A. Modulation of immunity and inflammatory gene expression in the gut, in inflammatory diseases of the gut and in the liver by probiotics. *World J Gastroenterol*. 2014;20(42):15632-15649.

[16] O'Mahony SM, Clarke G, Borre YE, Dinan TG, Cryan JF. Serotonin, tryptophan metabolism and the brain-gut-microbiome axis. *Behav Brain Res*. 2015;277:32-48. doi:10.1016/j.bbr.2014.07.027

[17] Ornish D, Ornish A. *Undo It!: How Simple Lifestyle Changes Can Reverse Most Chronic Diseases*. New York: Ballantine Books; 2019.

[18] Li WW. *Eat to Beat Disease: the New Science of How the Body Can Heal Itself.* New York: Grand Central Publishing; 2019.

[19] John Travis, "On the Origin of the Immune System," *Science* 324, no. 5927 (2009): 580-582, http://science.sciencemag.org/content/324/5927/580.

[20] B. Alberts et al., "B Cells and Antibodies," in *Molecular Biology of the Cell*, 4th ed. (New York: Garland Science, 2002). https://www,ncbi.nlm.nih.gov/books/NBK26884.

[21] L. A. DiPietro, "Angiogenesis and Wound Repair: When Enough is Enough," *Journal of Leukocyte Biology* 100, no. 5 (2016): 979-984.

[22] M. A. Gimbrone, S. B. Leapman, R. S. Cotran, and J. Folkman, "Tumor Dormancy In Vivo by Prevention of Neovascularization," *Journal of Experimental Medicine* 320, no. 18 (1989): 1197-1200.

[23] A. Albini et al., "Cancer Prevention by Targeting Angiogenesis," *Nature Reviews Clinical Oncology* 9, no. 9 (2012): 498-509.

[24] Milo R, Philips R. " How quickly do different cells in the body replace themselves? Cell biology by the numbers How quickly do different cells in the body replace themselves Comments. http://book.bionumbers.org/how-quickly-do-different-cells-in-the-body-replace-themselves/. Accessed March 29, 2020.

[25] B.N. Ames, M.K. Shigenaga, and T.M. Hagen, "Oxidants, Antioxidants, and the Degenerative Diseases of Aging."

[26] B. N. Ames, M. K. Shigenaga, and T. M. Hagen, "Oxidants, Antioxidants, and the Degenerative Disease of Aging," *Proceedings from the National Academy of Sciences USA* 90, no. 17 (1993): 7915-7922.

[27] Rizvi S, Raza ST, Mahdi F. Telomere length variations in aging and age-related diseases. *Curr Aging Sci.* 2014;7(3):161-167. doi:10.2174/1874609808666150122153151

[28] Stephen P. Jackson and Jiri Bartek, "The DNA-Damage Response in Human Biology and Disease," *nature* 461, no. 7267 (2009): 1071-1078.

[29] Liska DJ. The detoxification enzyme systems. *Altern Med Rev.* 1998;3(3);187-198

[30] Sapolsky RM. *Why Zebras Dont Get Ulcers: the Acclaimed Guide to Stress, Stress-Related Diseases, and Coping.* New York: Henry Holt and Co.; 2004.

[31] Buettner D. *The Blue Zones: 9 Lessons for Living Longer from the People Whove Lived the Longest.* Washington, D.C.: National Geographic; 2012.

[32] Buettner D. *The Blue Zones: 9 Lessons for Living Longer from the People Whove Lived the Longest.* Washington, D.C.: National Geographic; 2012.

[33] Hyman M. drmarkhyman.com. *drmarkhymancom.* https://drhyman.com/blog/2019/07/31/podcast-ep65/. Accessed March 11, 2020.

[34] Buettner D. *The Blue Zones: 9 Lessons for Living Longer from the People Whove Lived the Longest.* Washington, D.C.: National Geographic; 2012.

[35] Li WW. *Eat to Beat Disease: The New Science of How the Body Can Heal Itself.* New York: Grand Central Publishing; 2019.

[36] Domínguez R, Cuenca E, Maté-Muñoz JL, et al. Effects of Beetroot Juice Supplementation on Cardiorespiratory Endurance in Athletes. A Systematic Review. *Nutrients.* 2017;9(1):43. Published 2017 Jan 6. doi:10.3390/nu9010043

[37] Wightman EL, Haskell-Ramsay CF, Thompson KG, et al. Dietary nitrate modulates cerebral blood flow parameters and cognitive

performance in humans: A double-blind, placebo-controlled, crossover investigation. *Physiol Behav.* 2015;149:149-158. doi:10.1016/j.physbeh.2015.05.035

[38] Morris MC, Wang Y, Barnes LL, Bennett DA, Dawson-Hughes B, Booth SL. Nutrients and bioactives in green leafy vegetables and cognitive decline. *Neurology.* 2017;90(3). doi:10.1212/wnl.0000000000004815.

[39] Tucker KL, Hannan MT, Chen H, Cupples LA, Wilson PW, Kiel DP. Potassium, magnesium, and fruit and vegetable intakes are associated with greater bone mineral density in elderly men and women. *Am J Clin Nutr.* 1999;69(4):727-736. doi:10.1093/ajcn/69.4.727

[40] Makki K, Deehan EC, Walter J, Bäckhed F. The Impact of Dietary Fiber on Gut Microbiota in Host Health and Disease. *Cell Host Microbe.* 2018;23(6):705-715. doi:10.1016/j.chom.2018.05.012

[41] Holscher HD. Dietary fiber and prebiotics and the gastrointestinal microbiota. *Gut Microbes.* 2017;8(2):172-184. doi:10.1080/19490976.2017.1290756

[42] Hiel S, Bindels LB, Pachikian BD, et al. Effects of a diet based on inulin-rich vegetables on gut health and nutritional behavior in healthy humans. *Am J Clin Nutr.* 2019;109(6):1683-1695. doi:10.1093/ajcn/nqz001

[43] Le Bastard Q, Chapelet G, Javaudin F, Lepelletier D, Batard E, Montassier E. The effects of inulin on gut microbial composition: a systematic review of evidence from human studies. *Eur J Clin Microbiol Infect Dis.* 2020;39(3):403-413. doi:10.1007/s10096-019-03721-w

[44] Pacheco-Cano RD, Salcedo-Hernández R, López-Meza JE, Bideshi DK, Barboza-Corona JE. Antimicrobial activity of broccoli (Brassica oleracea var. italica) cultivar Avenger against pathogenic bacteria, phytopathogenic filamentous fungi and yeast. *J Appl Microbiol.* 2018;124(1):126-135. doi:10.1111/jam.13629

[45] Hosseini B, Berthon BS, Saedisomeolia A, et al. Effects of fruit and vegetable consumption on inflammatory biomarkers and immune cell populations: a systematic literature review and meta-analysis. *Am J Clin Nutr.* 2018;108(1):136-155. doi:10.1093/ajcn/nqy082

[46] M. P. Nantz et al., "Supplementation with Aged Garlic Improves Both NK and ydelta-T Cell Function and reduces the severity of Cold and Flu Symptoms: A Randomized, Double Blind, Placebo-Controlled Nutrition Intervention," *Clinical Nutrition* 31, no. 3 (2012): 337-344)

[47] J. W. Fahey, Y. Zhang, and P. Talalay, "broccoli Sprouts: An Exceptionally Rich Source of Inducers of Enzymes that Protect against Chemical Carcinogens," *Proceedings of the National Academy of Sciences USA* 94, no. 19 (1997): 10367-10372.

[48] H. Ishikawa et al., "Aged Garlic Extract Prevents a Decline of NK Cell Number and Activity in Patients with Advanced Cancer," *Journal of Nutrition* 136, no. 3, suppl. (2006): 816S-820S.

[49] R. Yu, J. W. Park, T. Kurata, and K. L. Erickson, " Modulation of Select Immune Responses to Dietary Capsaicin," *International Journal for Vitamin and Nutrition Research* 68, no. 2 (1998): 114-119

[50] J. Hendricks, C. Hoffman, D. W. Pascual, and M. E. Hardy, "18b-Glycyrrhetinic Acxid Delivered Orally Induces Isolated Lymphoid Follicle Maturation at the Intestinal Mucosa and Attenuates Rotavirus Shedding," PLOS One 7, no. 11 (2012): e49491)

[51] Baj T, Seth R. Role of Curcumin in Regulation of TNF-α Mediated Brain Inflammatory Responses. *Recent Pat Inflamm Allergy Drug Discov.* 2018;12(1):69-77. doi:10.2174/1872213X12666180703163824

[52] R. Liu et al., "Lutein and Zeaxanthin Supplementation and Association

with Visual Function in Age-related Macular Degeneration," Investigative Opthalmology and Visual Science 56, no. 1 (2014): 252-258

53 Li WW. *Eat to Beat Disease: The New Science of How the Body Can Heal Itself*. New York: Grand Central Publishing; 2019.

54 T. Kayashima and K. Matsubara, "Antiangiogenic Effect of Carnosic Acid and Carnosol, Neuroprotective Coumpouns in Rosemary Leaves," *Bioscience, Biotechnology, and Biochemistry* 76, no. 1 (2012): 115-119.

55 M. Saberi-Karimian et al., "Vascular Endothelial Growth Factor: An Important Molecular Target of Curcumin," *Critical Reviews in Food Science and Nutrition* (2017): 1-14.

56 P. Kubatka et al., "Oregano Demonstrates Distinct Tumour-Suppressive Effects in Breast Carcinoma Model," *European Journal of Nutrition* 56, no. 3 (2017): 1303-1316.

57 S. Kobayashi, T. Miyamoto, I. Kimura, and M. Kimura, "Inhibitory Effect of Isoliquiritin, a Compound in Licorice Root, on Angiogenesis In Vivo and Tube Formation In Vitro," *Biological and Pharmaceutical Bulletin* 18, no. 10 (1995): 1382-1386.

58 J. Lu et al. "Novel Angiogenesis Inhibitory Activity in Cinnamon Extract Blocks VEGFR2 Kinase and Downstream Signaling," *Carcinogenesis* 31, no. 3 (2010): 481-488.

59 M. Traka et al., "Transcriptome Analysis of Human Colon Caco-2 Cells Exposed to Sulforaphane," *Journal of Nutrition* 9, no. 1 (2007): R20) and increase tumor suppressor genes

60 Jiang A, Wang X, Shan X, et al. Curcumin Reactivates Silenced Tumor Suppressor Gene RARβ by Reducing DNA Methylation. *Phytother Res*. 2015;29(8):1237-1245. doi:10.1002/ptr.5373

61 R. Liu et al., "Lutein and Zeaxanthin Supplementation and Association with Visual Function in Age-related Macular Degeneration," Investigative Opthalmology and Visual Science 56, no. 1 (2014): 252-258

62 J. You et. al., "Curcumin Induces Therapeutic Angiogenesis in Diabetic Mouse Hindlimb Ischemia Model via Modulating the Function of Endothelial Progenitor Cell," *Stem Cell Research and Therapy* 8, no. 1 (2017): 182.)

63 The Detox Food Plan: IFM. The Institute for Functional Medicine. https://www.ifm.org/news-insights/detox-food-plan/. Accessed May 15, 2020.

64 Aga M, Iwaki K, Ueda Y, et al. Preventive effect of Coriandrum sativum (Chinese parsley) on localized lead deposition in ICR mice. *J Ethnopharmacol*. 2001;77(2-3):203-208.

65 Pollan M. *The Omnivores Dilemma: Young Readers Edition*. Turtleback Books; 2015.

66 Gerster H. Can adults adequately convert alpha-linolenic acid (18:3n-3) to eicosapentaenoic acid (20:5n-3) and docosahexaenoic acid (22:6n-3)?. *Int J Vitam Nutr Res*. 1998;68(3):159–173.

67 Huma, N., Anjum, M., Sehar, S., Issa Khan, M. and Hussain, S. (2008), "Effect of soaking and cooking on nutritional quality and safety of legumes", *Nutrition & Food Science*, Vol. 38 No. 6, pp. 570-577. https://doi.org/10.1108/00346650810920187

68 Okhonlaye O, Temitope O. Effect of Fermentation and Extrusion on the Nutrient and Anti-nutrient Composition of Soy Beans (Glycine max, L) and Acha (Digitaria exilis Stapf). *Microbiology Research Journal International*. 2017;21(1):1-21. doi:10.9734/mrji/2017/33263.

69 Sumiyoshi E, Matsuzaki K, Sugimoto N, et al. Sub-Chronic Consumption of Dark Chocolate Enhances Cognitive Function and Releases

Nerve Growth Factors: A Parallel-Group Randomized Trial. *Nutrients*. 2019;11(11):2800. Published 2019 Nov 16. doi:10.3390/nu11112800

[70] Arjmandi BH, Johnson SA, Pourafshar S, et al. Bone-Protective Effects of Dried Plum in Postmenopausal Women: Efficacy and Possible Mechanisms. *Nutrients*. 2017;9(5):496. Published 2017 May 14. doi:10.3390/nu9050496

[71] Fraga CG , Croft KD , Kennedy DO , Tomás-Barberán FA . The effects of polyphenols and other bioactives on human health. *Food Funct*. 2019;10(2):514-528. doi:10.1039/c8fo01997e

[72] Y. K. Lee et al., "Kiwifruit (*Actinidia deliciosa*) Changes Intestinal Microbial Profile," *Microbial Ecology in Health and Disease* 23 (2012).

[73] F. P. Martin et al., "Metabolic Effects of Dark Chocolate Consumption on Energy, Gut Microbiots, and Stress-Related Metabolism in Free-Living Subjects," *Journal of Proteome Research* 8, no. 12 (2009): 5568-5579.

[74] S. M. Henning et al., "Pomegranate ellagitannins Stimulate the Growth of Akkermansia municiphilia *In Vivo*," *Anaerobe* 43 (2017): 56-60.

[75] F. F. Anhe et al., "A Polyphenol-Rich Cranberry Extract Protects from DietOinduced Obesity, Insulin Resistance, and Intestinal Inflammation in Association with Increased *Akkermansia* spp. Population in the Gut Microbiota of Mice," *Gut* 64, no. 6 (2015): 872-883.

[76] C. Ceci et al., "Ellagic Acid Inhibits Bladder Cancer Invasiveness and In Vivo Tumor Growth," *Nutrients* 8, no. 11 (2016).

[77] S. J. Padayatty et al., "Vitamin C as an Antioxidant: Evaluation of Its Role in Disease Prevention," *Journal of the American College of Nutrition* 22, no. 1 (2003): 18-35

[78] A. R. Nair, N. Mariappan, A. J. Stull, and J. Francis, "Blueberry Supplementation Attenuates Oxidative Stress within Monocytes and Modulates Immune Cell Levels in Adults with Metabolic Syndrome: A Randomized, Double Blind, Placebo-Controlled Trial," *Food and Function* 8, no. 11 (2017): 5118-4128.

[79] L. S. McAnulty et al., "Effect of Blueberry Ingestion on Natural Killer Cell Counts, Oxidative Stress, and Inflammation prior to and after 2.5 h of Running," *Applied Physiology, Nutrition, and Metabolism* 36, no. 6 (2011): 976-984.

[80] M. Sumi et al., "Ursolic Acid and Ursolic Acid in Commercial Dried Fruits," *Food Science and Technology Research* 19, no. 1 (2013: 113-116.

[81] A. K. Maurya and M. Vinayak, "Quercetin Attenuates Cell Survival, Inflammation, and Angiogenesis via Modulation of AKT Signaling in Murine T-Cell Lymphoma," *Nutrition and Cancer* 69, no. 3 (2017): 470-480.

[82] S. Lamy et al., "Delphinidin, a Dietary Anthocyanidin, Inhibits Vascular Endothelial Growth Factor Receptor-2 Phosphorylatio," *Cardiogenesis* 27, no. 5 (2006): 989-996.

[83] R. E. Graff et al., "Dietary Lycopene Intake and Risk of Prostate Cancer Defined by ERG Protein Expression," *American Journal of Clinical Nutrition* 103, no. 3 (2016): 851-860.

[84] Rehman AUR. Effect of Cherry Juice on Angiogenesis Determined By Chorioallantoic Membrane (Cam) Assay. Austin J Nutr Metab. 2015; 2(5): 1032.

[85] T. P. Kenny et al., "Cocoa Procyanidins Inhibit Proliferation and Angiogenic Signals in Human Dermal Microvascular Endothetlial Cells following Stimulation by Low-Level H2O2," *Experimental Biology and Medicine* 229, no. 8 (2004): 765-771.

[86] A. Gajowik and M. M. Dobrzynska, "The Evaluation of Protective Effect of Lycopene against Genotoxic Influence of X-Irradiation in Human

Blood Lymphocytes," *Radiation and Environmental Biophysics* 56, no. 4 (2017): 413-422.

[87] J. K. Y. Hooi et al., "Global Prevelence of *Helicobacter pylori* Infection: Systematic Review and Meta-Analysis," *Gastroenterology* 153, no. 2 (2017): 420-429.

[88] A. R. Collins, V. Harrington, J. Drew, And R. Melvin, "Nutitional Modulation of DNA Repair in Human Intervention Study," *Carcinogenesis* 24, no. 3 (2003): 511-515.

[89] L.-S. Wang et. al., "Abstract 163: Metabolomic Profiling Reveals a Protective Modulation on Fatty Acid Metabolism in Colorectal Cancer Patients following Consumption of Freeze-Dried Black Raspberries," *Cancer Research* 73 (2013): 163

[90] J.H. An et al., "Effect of *Rubus occidentalis* Extract on Metabolic Parameters in Subjects with Prediabetes: A Proof-of-Concept, Randomized, Double Blind, Placebo-Controlled Clinical Trial," *Phytotherapy Research* 30, no. 10 (2016): 1634-1640

[91] L. Dugo et al., "Effect of Cocoa Polyphenolic Extract on Macrophage Polarization from Proinflammatory M1 to Anti-Inflammatory M2 State," *Oxidative Medicine and Cellular Longevity* 2017 (2017): 6293740.

[92] Gorbunov N, Petrovski G, Gurusamy N, Ray D, Kim DH, Das DK. Regeneration of infarcted myocardium with resveratrol-modified cardiac stem cells. *J Cell Mol Med.* 2012;16(1):174-184. doi:10.1111/j.1582-4934.2011.01281.x

[93] S. Li, H. Bian et al., "Chlorogenic Acid Protects MSCs against Oxidative Stress by Altering FOXO Family Genes and Activating Intrinsic Pathway," *European Journal of Pharmacology* 674, no. 2-3 (2012): 65-72

[94] Q. Deng, Y. X. Tian, and J. Liang, "Mangiferin Inhibits Cell Migration and Invasion through Racl/WAVE2 Signaling in Breast Cancer," *Cytotechnology* 70, no. 2 (2018): 593-601.

[95] M. Du et al., "Mangiferin Prevents the Growth of Gastric Carcinoma by Blocking the PI3K-Akt Signaling Pathway," *Anticancer Drugs* 29, no. 1 (2018): 167-175.

[96] H. L. Wang et al., "Mangiferin Facilitates Islet Regeneration and Beta-Cell Proliferation through Upregulation of Cell Cycle and Beta-Cell Regeneration Regulators," *International Journal of Molecular Sciences* 15, no. 5 (2014): 9016-9035.

[97] Y. Bai et al., "Mangiferin Enhances Endochondrial Ossification-Based Bone Repair in Massive Bone Defect by Inducing Autophagy through Activating AMP-Activated Protein Kinase Signaling Pathway," *FASEB Journal* 32, no. 8 (2018).

[98] S. J. Padayatty et al., "Vitamin C as an Antioxidant: Evaluation of Its Role in Disease Prevention," *Journal of the American College of Nutrition* 22, no. 1 (2003): 18-35

[99] Fox M, Meyer-Gerspach AC, Wendebourg MJ, et al. Effect of cocoa on the brain and gut in healthy subjects: a randomised controlled trial. *Br J Nutr.* 2019;121(6):654-661. doi:10.1017/S0007114518003689

[100] The Detox Food Plan: IFM. The Institute for Functional Medicine. https://www.ifm.org/news-insights/detox-food-plan/. Accessed June 14, 2020.

[101] Kuebler U, Arpagaus A, Meister RE, et al. Dark chocolate attenuates intracellular pro-inflammatory reactivity to acute psychosocial stress in men: A randomized controlled trial. *Brain Behav Immun.* 2016;57:200-208. doi:10.1016/j.bbi.2016.04.006

[102] Hoffman JR, Falvo MJ. Protein - Which is Best?. *J Sports Sci Med.* 2004;3(3):118-130. Published 2004 Sep 1.

[103] Hoffman JR, Falvo MJ. Protein - Which is Best?. *J Sports Sci Med.* 2004;3(3):118-130. Published 2004 Sep 1.

[104] Daley CA, Abbott A, Doyle PS, Nader GA, Larson S. A review of fatty acid profiles and antioxidant content in grass-fed and grain-fed beef. *Nutr J.* 2010;9:10. Published 2010 Mar 10. doi:10.1186/1475-2891-9-10

[105] D. J. Lisko, G. P. Johnston, and C. G. Johnston, "Effects of Dietary Yogurt on the Healthy Human Gastrointestinal (GI) Microbiome," *Microorganisms* 5, no. 1 (2017).

[106] K. Van Hoorde, M. Heyndrickx, P. Vandamme, and G. Huys, "Influence of Pasteurization, Brining Conditions, and Production Environment on the Microbiota of Artisan Gouda-Type Cheeses," *Food Microbiology* 27, no. 3 (2010): 425-433.

[107] Zaheer, K. (2015) An Updated Review on Chicken Eggs: Production, Consumption, Management Aspects and Nutritional Benefits to Human Health. *Food and Nutrition Sciences,* 6, 1208-1220. doi: 10.4236/fns.2015.613127.

[108] Andersen CJ. Bioactive Egg Components and Inflammation. *Nutrients.* 2015;7(9):7889-7913. Published 2015 Sep 16. doi:10.3390/nu7095372

[109] Rennard BO, Ertl RF, Gossman GL, Robbins RA, Rennard SI. Chicken Soup Inhibits Neutrophil Chemotaxis In Vitro. *Chest.* 2000;118(4):1150-1157. doi:10.1378/chest.118.4.1150.

[110] T. J. Koivu-Tikkanen, V. Ollilainen, and V. I. Piironen, "Determination of Phylloquinone and Menaquinones in Animal Products with Fluorescence Detection after Postcolumn Reduction with Metallic Zinc," *Journal of Agricultural and Food Chemistry* 48, no. 12 (2000): 6325-6331.

[111] T. J. Koivu-Tikkanen, V. Ollilainen, and V. I. Piironen, "Determination of Phylloquinone and Menaquinones in Animal Products with Fluorescence Detection after Postcolumn Reduction with Metallic Zinc," *Journal of Agricultural and Food Chemistry* 48, no. 12 (2000): 6325-6331.

[112] C. Vermeer et al., "menaquinone Content of Cheese," *Nutrients* 10, no. 4 (2018).

[113] Fretts AM, Howard BV, Siscovick DS, et al. Processed Meat, but Not Unprocessed Red Meat, Is Inversely Associated with Leukocyte Telomere Length in the Strong Heart Family Study. *J Nutr.* 2016;146(10):2013-2018. doi:10.3945/jn.116.234922

[114] Kasielski M, Eusebio MO, Pietruczuk M, Nowak D. The relationship between peripheral blood mononuclear cells telomere length and diet - unexpected effect of red meat. *Nutr J.* 2016;15(1):68. Published 2016 Jul 14. doi:10.1186/s12937-016-0189-2

[115] Mazucanti CH, Cabral-Costa JV, Vasconcelos AR, Andreotti DZ, Scavone C, Kawamoto EM. Longevity Pathways (mTOR, SIRT, Insulin/IGF-1) as Key Modulatory Targets on Aging and Neurodegeneration. *Curr Top Med Chem.* 2015;15(21):2116-2138. doi:10.2174/1568026615666150610125715

[116] Weichhart T. mTOR as Regulator of Lifespan, Aging, and Cellular Senescence: A Mini-Review. *Gerontology.* 2018;64(2):127-134. doi:10.1159/000484629

[117] Li W. Eggs: Health Food or Best Avoided? Dr William Li. https://drwilliamli.com/eggs-healthy-or-unhealthy/. Published April 23, 2019. Accessed March 14, 2020.

[118] Beuttner, D., 2020. *Food Guidelines - Blue Zones.* [online] Blue Zones. Available at: <https://www.bluezones.com/recipes/food-guidelines/> [Accessed 14 March 2020].

[119] Brannon PM, Carpenter TO, Fernandez JR, Gilsanz V, Gould JB, Hall KE, Hui SL, Lupton JR, Mennella J, Miller NJ, Osganian SK, Sellmeyer DE, Suchy FJ, Wolf MA. NIH Consensus Development Conference Statement: Lactose Intolerance and Health. NIH Consens State Sci Statements. 2010 Feb 24;27(2).

[120] Uribarri J, Woodruff S, Goodman S, et al. Advanced Glycation End Products in Foods and a Practical Guide to Their Reduction in the Diet. *Journal of the American Dietetic Association.* 2010;110(6). doi:10.1016/j.jada.2010.03.018.

[121] Andruchow ND, Konishi K, Shatenstein B, Bohbot VD. A lower ratio of omega-6 to omega-3 fatty acids predicts better hippocampus-dependent spatial memory and cognitive status in older adults. *Neuropsychology.* 2017;31(7):724-734. doi:10.1037/neu0000373

[122] D. Mozaffarian et al., "Plasma Phospholipid Long-Chain omega-3 Fatty Acids and Total and Cause-specific Mortality in Older Adults: A Cohort Study," *Annals of Internal Medicine* 158, no. 7 (2013): 515-525.

[123] Costantini L, Molinari R, Farinon B, Merendino N. Impact of Omega-3 Fatty Acids on the Gut Microbiota. *Int J Mol Sci.* 2017;18(12):2645. Published 2017 Dec 7. doi:10.3390/ijms18122645

[124] J. Y. Cheng, L. T. Ng, C. L. Lin, and T. R. Jan, "Pacific Oyster-Derived Polysaccharides Enhance Antigen-Specific T Helper (Th)1 Immunity In Vitro and In Vivo," *Immunopharmacology and Immunotoxicology* 35, no. 2 (2013): 235-240.

[125] S. A. Messina and R. Dawson Jr., "Attenuation of Oxidative Damage to DNA by Taurine and Taurine Analogs," *Advances in Experimental Medicine and Biology* 483 (2000): 355-367

[126] Calder PC. Omega-3 fatty acids and inflammatory processes: from molecules to man. *Biochem Soc Trans.* 2017;45(5):1105-1115. doi:10.1042/BST20160474

[127] Block RC, Dier U, Calderonartero P, et al. The Effects of EPA+DHA and Aspirin on Inflammatory Cytokines and Angiogenesis Factors. *World J Cardiovasc Dis.* 2012;2(1):14-19. doi:10.4236/wjcd.2012.21003

[128] C. Sakai et al., "Fish Oil Omega-3 Polyunsaturated Fatty Acids Attenuate Oxidative Stress-Induced DNA Damage in Vascular Endothelial Cells," *PLOS One* 12, no. 11 (2017): e0187934.

[129] J. Turgeon et al., "Fish Oil-Enriched Diet Protects against Ischemia by Improving Angiogenesis, Endothelial Progenitor Cell Function, and Postnatal Neovascularization," *Atherosclerosis* 229, no. 2 (2013):295-303.

[130] Delarue,J, Matzinger O, Binnert C, et al. Fish oil prevents the adrenal activation elicited by mental stress in healthy men. Diabetes Metab 2003;29:289-295.

[131] W. G. Christen et al., "Dietary Omega-3 Fatty Acid and Fish Intake and Incident Age-Related Macular Degeneration in Women," *Archives of Opthalmology* 129, no. 7 (2011): 921-929.

[132] Del Gobbo LC, Falk MC, Feldman R, Lewis K, Mozaffarian D. Effects of tree nuts on blood lipids, apolipoproteins, and blood pressure: systematic review, meta-analysis, and dose-response of 61 controlled intervention trials. *Am J Clin Nutr.* 2015;102(6):1347-1356. doi:10.3945/ajcn.115.110965

[133] Bourre, J.M. Brain lipids and aging. In: *For the Ageing Population.* Woodhead Publishing Limited; 2009:219-251. https://www.sciencedirect.com/science/article/pii/B9781845691936500129. Accessed April 9, 2020.

[134] C. Bamberger et al., "A Walnut-Enriched Diet Affects Gut Microbiome in Healthy Caucasian Subjects: A Randomized, Controlled Trial," *Nutrients* 10, no. 2 (2018).

[135] Ros E. Health benefits of nut consumption. *Nutrients.* 2010;2(7):652-682. doi:10.3390/nu2070652

[136] Majdalawieh AF, Massri M, Nasrallah GK. A comprehensive review on the anti-cancer properties and mechanisms of action of sesamin, a lignan in sesame seeds (Sesamum indicum). *Eur J Pharmacol.* 2017;815:512-521. doi:10.1016/j.ejphar.2017.10.020

[137] Li WW. *Eat to Beat Disease: the New Science of How the Body Can Heal Itself.* New York: Grand Central Publishing; 2019.

[138] J. X. Kang and A. Liu, "The Role of the Tissue Omega-6/Omega-3 Fatty Acid Ratio in Regulating Tumor Angiogenesis," *Cancer and Metastasis Reviews* 32, no. 1-2 (2013): 201-210.

[139] Tucker LA. Consumption of Nuts and Seeds and Telomere Length in 5,582 Men and Women of the National Health and Nutrition Examination Survey (NHANES). *J Nutr Health Aging.* 2017;21(3):233-240. doi:10.1007/s12603-017-0876-5

[140] Ling L, Gu S, Cheng Y. Resveratrol activates endogenous cardiac stem cells and improves myocardial regeneration following acute myocardial infarction. *Mol Med Rep.* 2017;15(3):1188-1194. doi:10.3892/mmr.2017.6143

[141] Liu QS, Li SR, Li K, Li X, Yin X, Pang Z. Ellagic acid improves endogenous neural stem cells proliferation and neurorestoration through Wnt/β-catenin signaling in vivo and in vitro. *Mol Nutr Food Res.* 2017;61(3):10.1002/mnfr.201600587. doi:10.1002/mnfr.201600587

[142] J. M. Monk et al., "Navy and Black Bean Supplementation Primes the Colonic Mucosal Microenvironment to Improve Gut Health," *Journal of Nutritional Biochemistry* 49 (2017): 89-100.

[143] J. M. Monk et al., "Navy and Black Bean Supplementation Primes the Colonic Mucosal Microenvironment to Improve Gut Health," *Journal of Nutritional Biochemistry* 49 (2017): 89-100.

[144] Zhu F, Du B, Xu B. Anti-inflammatory effects of phytochemicals from fruits, vegetables, and food legumes: A review. *Crit Rev Food Sci Nutr.* 2018;58(8):1260-1270. doi:10.1080/10408398.2016.1251390

[145] T. Fotsis et al., "Genistein, a Dietary-derived Inhibito of Vitro Angiogenesis," *Proceedings of the National Academy of Sciences USA* 90, no. 7 suppl. (1993): 2690-2694.

[146] S. H. Lee, J. Lee, M. H. Jung, and Y. M. Lee, "Glyceollins, a Novel Class of Soy Phytoalexins, Inhibit Angiogenesis by Blocking the VEGF and bFGF Signaling Pathways," *Molecular Nutrition and Food Research* 57, no. 2 (2013): 225-234.

[147] M. Z. Fang et al., "Reversal of Hypermethylation and Reactivation pf p16INK4a, RARbeta, and MGMT Genes by Genistein and Other Isoflavones from Soy," *Clinical Cancer Research* 11, no. 19, pt. 1 (2005): 7033-7041.

[148] X. O. Shu et al., "Soy Food Intake and Breast Cancer Survival," *JAMA* 302, no. 22 (2009): 2437-2443.

[149] C. C. Applegate et al., "Soy Consumption and the Risk of Prostate Cancer: An Updated Systematic Review and Meta-Analysis," *Nutrients* 10, no. 1 (2018)

[150] Margier M, Georgé S, Hafnaoui N, et al. Nutritional Composition and Bioactive Content of Legumes: Characterization of Pulses Frequently Consumed in France and Effect of the Cooking Method. *Nutrients.* 2018;10(11):1668. Published 2018 Nov 4. doi:10.3390/nu10111668

[151] Hoffman JR, Falvo MJ. Protein - Which is Best?. *J Sports Sci Med.* 2004;3(3):118-130. Published 2004 Sep 1.

[152] Huma, N., Anjum, M., Sehar, S., Issa Khan, M. and Hussain, S. (2008), "Effect of soaking and cooking on nutritional quality and safety of legumes", *Nutrition & Food Science*, Vol. 38 No. 6, pp. 570-577. https://doi.org/10.1108/00346650810920187

[153] S. Lecomte, F. Demay, F Ferriere, and F. Pakdel, "Phytochemicals Targetinf Estrogen Receptors: Beneficial Rather than Adverse Effects?" *International Journal of Molecular Sciences* 18, no.7 (2017): E1381.

[154] Cardwell G, Bornman JF, James AP, Black LJ. A Review of Mushrooms as a Potential Source of Dietary Vitamin D. *Nutrients.* 2018;10(10):1498. Published 2018 Oct 13. doi:10.3390/nu10101498

[155] X. Jiang et al., "The Anti-Fatigue Activities of Tubor Melanosporum in a Mouse Model," *Experimental and Therapeutic Medicine* 15, no. 3 (2018): 3066-3074

[156] W. Rssouw and L. Korsten, "Cultivable Microbiome of Fresh White Button Mushrooms," *Letters in Applied Microbiology* 64, no. 2 (2017): 164-170.

[157] J. Varshney et al., "White Button Mushrooms Increase Microbial Diversity and Accelerate the Resolution of *Citrobacter rodentium* Infection in Mice," *Journal of Nutrition* 143, no. 4 (2013): 526-532.

[158] S. C. Jeong, S. R. Koyyalamudi, and G. Pang, "Dietary Intake of *Agaricus bisporus* White Button Mushroom Accelerates Salivary Immunoglobulin A Secretion in Healthy Volunteers," *Nutrition* 28, no. 5 (2010): 527-531.

[159] K. I. Minato, L. C. Laan, A. Ohara, and I. can Die, "Pleurotus Citrinopileatus Polysaccharide Induces Activation of Human Dendritic Cells through Multiple Pathways," *International Immunopharmacology* 40 (2016): 156-163.

[160] H. H. Chang et al., "Oral Administration of an Enoki Mushroom Protein FVE Activates Innate and Adaptive Immunity and Induces Anti-tumor Activity against Murine Hepatocellular Carcinoma," *International Immunopharmacology* 10, no. 2 (2010): 239-246.

[161] V. Vetcicka and J. Vetvickova, "Immune-Enhancing Effects of Maitake (*Grifola frondosa*) and Shiitake (*Lentinula edodes*) Extracts," *Annals of Translational Medicine* 2, no. 2 (2014): 14.

[162] G. Pacioni et al., "Truffles Contain Endocannabinoid Metabolic Enzymes and Anandamide," *Phytochemistry* 110 (2015): 104-110

[163] N. Acharya et al., "Endocannabinoid System Acts as a Regulator of Immune Homeostasis in the Gut," *Proceedings of the National Academy of Sciences USA* 114, no. 19 (2017): 5005-5010

[164] B. M. Fonseca, G. Correia-Da-Sylva, and N. A. Teixiera, "Cannabinoid-Induced Cell Death in Endometrial Cancer Cells: Involvement of TRPV1 Receptors in Apoptosis," *Journal of Physiology and Biochemistry* 74, no. 2 (2018)

[165] X. Jiang et al., "The Anti-Fatigue Activities of Tubor Melanosporum in a Mouse Model," *Experimental and Therapeutic Medicine* 15, no. 3 (2018): 3066-3074

[166] Erdman SE, Poutahidis T. Probiotic 'glow of health': it's more than skin deep. *Benef Microbes.* 2014;5(2):109-119. doi:10.3920/BM2013.0042

[167] Park KY, Jeong JK, Lee YE, Daily JW 3rd. Health benefits of kimchi (Korean fermented vegetables) as a probiotic food. *J Med Food.* 2014;17(1):6-20. doi:10.1089/jmf.2013.3083

[168] Homayoni Rad A, Vaghef Mehrabany E, Alipoor B, Vaghef Mehrabany L. The Comparison of Food and Supplement as Probiotic Delivery Vehicles. *Crit Rev Food Sci Nutr.* 2016;56(6):896-909. doi:10.1080/10408398.2012.733894

[169] Poutahidis T, Kearney SM, Levkovich T, et al. Microbial symbionts accelerate wound healing via the neuropeptide hormone oxytocin. *PLoS One.* 2013;8(10):e78898. Published 2013 Oct 30. doi:10.1371/journal.pone.0078898

[170] Athiyyah AF, Darma A, Ranuh R, et al. Lactobacillus plantarum IS-10506 activates intestinal stem cells in a rodent model. *Benef Microbes.* 2018;9(5):755-760. doi:10.3920/BM2017.0118

[171] Poutahidis T, Kearney SM, Levkovich T, et al. Microbial symbionts accelerate wound healing via the neuropeptide hormone oxytocin. *PLoS One.* 2013;8(10):e78898. Published 2013 Oct 30. doi:10.1371/journal.pone.0078898

[172] Thomson AB, Keelan M, Garg M, Clandinin MT. Dietary effects of omega 3-fatty acids on intestinal transport function. *Can J Physiol Pharmacol.* 1988;66(8):985-992. doi:10.1139/y88-162

[173] Costantini L, Molinari R, Farinon B, Merendino N. Impact of Omega-3 Fatty Acids on the Gut Microbiota. *Int J Mol Sci.* 2017;18(12):2645. Published 2017 Dec 7. doi:10.3390/ijms18122645

[174] Teng M, Zhao YJ, Khoo AL, Yeo TC, Yong QW, Lim BP. Impact of coconut oil consumption on cardiovascular health: a systematic review and meta-analysis. *Nutr Rev.* 2020;78(3):249-259. doi:10.1093/nutrit/nuz074

[175] Melguizo-Rodríguez L, Manzano-Moreno FJ, Illescas-Montes R, et al. Bone Protective Effect of Extra-Virgin Olive Oil Phenolic Compounds by Modulating Osteoblast Gene Expression. *Nutrients.* 2019;11(8):1722. Published 2019 Jul 25. doi:10.3390/nu11081722

[176] Dupont J, Dedeyne L, Dalle S, Koppo K, Gielen E. The role of omega-3 in the prevention and treatment of sarcopenia. *Aging Clin Exp Res.* 2019;31(6):825-836. doi:10.1007/s40520-019-01146-1

[177] Costantini L, Molinari R, Farinon B, Merendino N. Impact of Omega-3 Fatty Acids on the Gut Microbiota. *Int J Mol Sci.* 2017;18(12):2645. Published 2017 Dec 7. doi:10.3390/ijms18122645

[178] Marcelino G, Hiane PA, Freitas KC, et al. Effects of Olive Oil and Its Minor Components on Cardiovascular Diseases, Inflammation, and Gut Microbiota. *Nutrients.* 2019;11(8):1826. Published 2019 Aug 7. doi:10.3390/nu11081826

[179] Aparicio-Soto M, Sánchéz-Hidalgo M, Cárdeno A, et al. The phenolic fraction of extra virgin olive oil modulates the activation and the inflammatory response of T cells from patients with systemic lupus erythematosus and healthy donors. *Mol Nutr Food Res.*

[180] Servili M, Sordini B, Esposto S, et al. Biological Activities of Phenolic Compounds of Extra Virgin Olive Oil. *Antioxidants (Basel).* 2013;3(1):1-23. Published 2013 Dec 20. doi:10.3390/antiox3010001

[181] Moosavian SP, Arab A, Mehrabani S, Moradi S, Nasirian M. The effect of omega-3 and vitamin E on oxidative stress and inflammation: Systematic review and meta-analysis of randomized controlled trials [published online ahead of print, 2019 Aug 23]. *Int J Vitam Nutr Res.* 2019;1-11. doi:10.1024/0300-9831/a000599

[182] Pupala SS, Rao S, Strunk T, Patole S. Topical application of coconut oil to the skin of preterm infants: a systematic review. *Eur J Pediatr.* 2019;178(9):1317-1324. doi:10.1007/s00431-019-03407-7

[183] Calabriso N, Massaro M, Scoditti E, et al. Extra virgin olive oil rich in polyphenols modulates VEGF-induced angiogenic responses by preventing NADPH oxidase activity and expression. *J Nutr Biochem.* 2016;28:19-29.

[184] A. P. Simopoulos, "The Importance of the Omega-6/Omega-3 Fatty Acid Ratio in Cardiovascular Disease and Other Chronic Diseases," *Experimental Biology and Medicine* 233, no. 6 (2008): 674-688.

[185] Cordero JG, García-Escudero R, Avila J, Gargini R, García-Escudero V. Benefit of Oleuropein Aglycone for Alzheimer's Disease by Promoting Autophagy. *Oxid Med Cell Longev.* 2018;2018:5010741. Published 2018 Feb 20. doi:10.1155/2018/5010741

[186] Rigacci S. Olive Oil Phenols as Promising Multi-targeting Agents Against Alzheimer's Disease. *Adv Exp Med Biol.* 2015;863:1-20. doi:10.1007/978-3-319-18365-7_1

[187] Barnard ND, Bunner AE, Agarwal U. Saturated and trans fats and dementia: a systematic review. *Neurobiol Aging.* 2014;35 Suppl 2:S65-S73. doi:10.1016/j.neurobiolaging.2014.02.030

[188] Soto-Alarcon SA, Valenzuela R, Valenzuela A, Videla LA. Liver Protective Effects of Extra Virgin Olive Oil: Interaction between Its Chemical Composition and the Cell-signaling Pathways Involved in Protection. *Endocr Metab Immune Disord Drug Targets.* 2018;18(1):75-84.

[189] Katina K, Arendt E, Liukkonen K-H, Autio K, Flander L, Poutanen K. Potential of sourdough for healthier cereal products. *Trends in Food Science & Technology.* 2005;16(1-3):104-112. doi:10.1016/j.tifs.2004.03.008.

[190] Q. Mu, V. J. Tavella, and X. M. Luo, "Role of *Lactobacillus reuteri* in Human Health and Diseases," *Frontiers in Microbiology* 9, no. 757 (2018).

[191] Cagno RD, Angelis MD, Auricchio S, et al. Sourdough Bread Made from Wheat and Nontoxic Flours and Started with Selected Lactobacilli Is Tolerated in Celiac Sprue Patients. *Applied and Environmental Microbiology.* 2004;70(2):1088-1096. doi:10.1128/aem.70.2.1088-1096.2004.

[192] J. R. Lakritz et al., "Beneficial Bacteria Stimulate Host Immune Cells to Counteract Dietary and Genetic Predisposition to Mammary Cancer in Mice," *International Journal of Cancer* 135, no. 3 (2014): 529-540.

[193] Coda R, Rizzello CG, Pinto D, Gobbetti M. Selected lactic acid bacteria synthesize antioxidant peptides during sourdough fermentation of cereal flours. *Appl Environ Microbiol.* 2012;78(4):1087-1096. doi:10.1128/AEM.06837-11

[194] Michalska A, Ceglinska A, Amarowicz R, Piskula MK, Szawara-Nowak D, Zielinski H. Antioxidant contents and antioxidative properties of traditional rye breads. *J Agric Food Chem.* 2007;55(3):734-740. doi:10.1021/jf062425w

[195] C. Perez-Ternero et al., "Ferulic Acid, a Bioactive Compound of Rice Bran, Improves Oxidative Stress and Mitochondrial Biogenesis and Dynamics in Mice and in Human Mononuclear Cells," *Journal of Nutritional Biochemistry* 48 (2017):51-61.

[196] Poutahidis T, Kearney SM, Levkovich T, et al. Microbial symbionts accelerate wound healing via the neuropeptide hormone oxytocin. *PLoS One.* 2013;8(10):e78898. Published 2013 Oct 30. doi:10.1371/journal.pone.0078898

[197] Davis W. *Wheat Belly: Lose the Wheat, Lose the Weight, and Find Your Path Back to Health.* New York: Rodale; 2019.

[198] Power 9®. Blue Zones. https://www.bluezones.com/2016/11/power-9/. Published June 2, 2020. Accessed June 20, 2020.

[199] Longo V. *The Longevity Diet: Slow Aging, Fight Disease, Optimize Weight.* New York: Avery, an imprint of Penguin Random House; 2019.

[200] Carmona JJ, Michan S. Biology of Healthy Aging and Longevity. *Rev Invest Clin.* 2016;68(1):7-16.

[201] Holderbaum M, Casagrande DS, Sussenbach S, Buss C. Effects of very low calorie diets on liver size and weight loss in the preoperative period of bariatric surgery: a systematic review. *Surg Obes Relat Dis.* 2018;14(2):237-244. doi:10.1016/j.soard.2017.09.531

[202] Cho Y, Hong N, Kim KW, et al. The Effectiveness of Intermittent Fasting to Reduce Body Mass Index and Glucose Metabolism: A Systematic Review and Meta-Analysis. *J Clin Med.* 2019;8(10):1645. Published 2019 Oct 9. doi:10.3390/jcm8101645

[203] Genton L, Cani P, Schrenzel J. Alterations of gut barrier and gut microbiota in food restriction, food deprivation and protein-energy wasting. *Clinical Nutrition.* 2015;34(3):341-349. doi:10.1016/j.clnu.2014.10.003.

[204] Aldewachi HS, Wright NA, Appleton DR, Watson AJ: The effect of starvation and refeeding on cell population kinetics in the rat small bowel mucosa. J Anat 119:105-121, 1975

[205] Christovam AC, Theodoro V, Mendonça FAS, Esquisatto MAM, Dos Santos GMT, do Amaral MEC. Activators of SIRT1 in wound repair: an animal model study. *Arch Dermatol Res.* 2019;311(3):193-201. doi:10.1007/s00403-019-01901-4

[206] M. Igarashi and L. Guarente, "mTORC1 and SIRT1 Cooperate to Foster Expansion of Gut Adult Stem Cells during Caloric Restriction," *Cell* 166, no. 2 (2016): 436-450

[207] Suzanne Wu, "Fasting Triggers Stem Cell Regeneration of Damaged, Old Immune System," USC New, June 5, 2014, https://news.usc.edu/63669/fasting -triggers-stem-cell-regeneration-of-damaged-old-immune-system.

[208] C. W. Cheng et al., "Prolonged Fasting Reduces IGF-1/PKA to Promote Hematopoietic-Stem-Cell-Based Regeneration and Reverse Immunosuppression," *Cell Stem Cell* 14, no.6 (2014): 810-823

[209] Bagheriya M, Butler AE, Barreto GE, Sahebkar A. The effect of fasting or calorie restriction on autophagy induction: A review of the literature. *Ageing Res Rev.* 2018;47:183-197. doi:10.1016/j.arr.2018.08.004

[210] Araya-Quintanilla F, Celis-Rosati A, Rodriguez-Leiva C, Silva-Navarro C, Silva-Pinto Y, Toro-Jeria B. Efectividad de la dieta cetogenica en niños con epilepsia refractaria: revision sistematica [Effectiveness of a ketogenic diet in children with refractory epilepsy: a systematic review]. *Rev Neurol.* 2016;62(10):439-448.

[211] Avgerinos KI, Egan JM, Mattson MP, Kapogiannis D. Medium Chain Triglycerides induce mild ketosis and may improve cognition in Alzheimer's disease. A systematic review and meta-analysis of human studies. *Ageing Res Rev.* 2020;58:101001. doi:10.1016/j.arr.2019.101001

[212] Castellana M, Conte E, Cignarelli A, et al. Efficacy and safety of very low calorie ketogenic diet (VLCKD) in patients with overweight and obesity: A systematic review and meta-analysis [published online ahead of print, 2019 Nov 9]. *Rev Endocr Metab Disord.* 2019;10.1007/s11154-019-09514-y. doi:10.1007/s11154-019-09514-y

[213] Fan Y, Wang H, Liu X, Zhang J, Liu G. Crosstalk between the Ketogenic Diet and Epilepsy: From the Perspective of Gut Microbiota. *Mediators Inflamm.* 2019;2019:8373060. Published 2019 Jun 3. doi:10.1155/2019/8373060

[214] Paoli A, Mancin L, Bianco A, Thomas E, Mota JF, Piccini F. Ketogenic Diet and Microbiota: Friends or Enemies?. *Genes (Basel).* 2019;10(7):534. Published 2019 Jul 15. doi:10.3390/genes10070534

215 Pinto A, Bonucci A, Maggi E, Corsi M, Businaro R. Anti-Oxidant and Anti-Inflammatory Activity of Ketogenic Diet: New Perspectives for Neuroprotection in Alzheimer's Disease. *Antioxidants (Basel)*. 2018;7(5):63. Published 2018 Apr 28. doi:10.3390/antiox7050063

216 Woolf EC, Syed N, Scheck AC. Tumor Metabolism, the Ketogenic Diet and β-Hydroxybutyrate: Novel Approaches to Adjuvant Brain Tumor Therapy. *Front Mol Neurosci*. 2016;9:122. Published 2016 Nov 16. doi:10.3389/fnmol.2016.00122

217 Paoli A, Mancin L, Bianco A, Thomas E, Mota JF, Piccini F. Ketogenic Diet and Microbiota: Friends or Enemies?. *Genes (Basel)*. 2019;10(7):534. Published 2019 Jul 15. doi:10.3390/genes10070534

218 Cheng CW, Biton M, Haber AL, et al. Ketone Body Signaling Mediates Intestinal Stem Cell Homeostasis and Adaptation to Diet. *Cell*. 2019;178(5):1115-1131.e15. doi:10.1016/j.cell.2019.07.048

219 Livingstone, M. Barbara E., and L. Kirsty Pourshahidi. "Portion size and obesity." *Advances in nutrition* 5.6 (2014): 829-834.

220 Lamming DW, Ye L, Sabatini DM, Baur JA. Rapalogs and mTOR inhibitors as anti-aging therapeutics. *J Clin Invest*. 2013;123(3):980-989. doi:10.1172/JCI64099

221 Lamming DW. Inhibition of the Mechanistic Target of Rapamycin (mTOR)-Rapamycin and Beyond. *Cold Spring Harb Perspect Med*. 2016;6(5):a025924. Published 2016 May 2. doi:10.1101/cshperspect.a025924

222 E. Y. Huang et al., "The Role of Diet in Triggering Human Inflammatory Disorders in the Modern Age," *Microbes and Infection* 15, no. 12 (2013): 765-774.

223 Gunnars K. How to Optimize Your Omega-6 to Omega-3 Ratio. Healthline. https://www.healthline.com/nutrition/optimize-omega-6-omega-3-ratio#section3. Accessed June 22, 2020.

224 Choo VL, Viguiliouk E, Blanco Mejia S, et al. Food sources of fructose-containing sugars and glycaemic control: systematic review and meta-analysis of controlled intervention studies [published correction appears in BMJ. 2019 Oct 9;367:l5524]. *BMJ*. 2018;363:k4644. Published 2018 Nov 21. doi:10.1136/bmj.k4644

225 DiNicolantonio JJ, O'Keefe JH, Wilson WL Sugar addiction: is it real? A narrative review *British Journal of Sports Medicine* 2018;52:910-913.

226 Van Name M, Giannini C, Santoro N, et al. Blunted suppression of acyl-ghrelin in response to fructose ingestion in obese adolescents: the role of insulin resistance. *Obesity (Silver Spring)*. 2015;23(3):653-661. doi:10.1002/oby.21019

227 Yau AM, McLaughlin J, Maughan RJ, Gilmore W, Evans GH. The Effect of Short-Term Dietary Fructose Supplementation on Gastric Emptying Rate and Gastrointestinal Hormone Responses in Healthy Men. *Nutrients*. 2017;9(3):258. Published 2017 Mar 10. doi:10.3390/nu9030258

228 Ter Horst KW, Serlie MJ. Fructose Consumption, Lipogenesis, and Non-Alcoholic Fatty Liver Disease. *Nutrients*. 2017;9(9):981. Published 2017 Sep 6. doi:10.3390/nu9090981

229 Spencer M, Gupta A, Dam LV, Shannon C, Menees S, Chey WD. Artificial Sweeteners: A Systematic Review and Primer for Gastroenterologists. *J Neurogastroenterol Motil*. 2016;22(2):168-180. doi:10.5056/jnm15206

230 Romo-Romo A, Aguilar-Salinas CA, Brito-Córdova GX, Gómez-Díaz RA, Almeda-Valdes P. Sucralose decreases insulin sensitivity in healthy

subjects: a randomized controlled trial. *Am J Clin Nutr.* 2018;108(3):485-491. doi:10.1093/ajcn/nqy152

231 Gugliucci A. Formation of Fructose-Mediated Advanced Glycation End Products and Their Roles in Metabolic and Inflammatory Diseases. *Adv Nutr.* 2017;8(1):54-62. Published 2017 Jan 17. doi:10.3945/an.116.013912

232 Aragno M, Mastrocola R. Dietary Sugars and Endogenous Formation of Advanced Glycation Endproducts: Emerging Mechanisms of Disease. *Nutrients.* 2017;9(4):385. Published 2017 Apr 14. doi:10.3390/nu9040385

233 C. W. Leung et al., "Soda and Cell Aging: Associations between Sugar-Sweetened Beverage Consumption and Leukocytetelomere Length in Healthy Adults from the National Health and Nutrition Examination Surveys," *American Journal of Public Health* 104, no. 12 (2014): 2425-2431

234 H. Kang et al., "High Glucose-Induced Endothelial Progenitor Cell Dysfunction," *Diabetes and Vascular Disease Research* 14, no. 5 (2017): 381-394

235 J. Wang et al., "High Glucose Inhibits Osteogenic Differentiation through the BMP Signaling Pathway in Bone Mesenchymal Cells in Mice," *EXCLI Journal* 12 (2013): 584-597

236 H. Y. Choi et al., " High Glucose Causes Human Cardiac Progenitor Cell Dysfunction by Promoting Mitochondrial Fission: Role of GLUT1 Blocker," *Biomolecules and Therapeuticsl* 24, no. 4 (2016): 363-370

237 Leech B, McIntyre E, Steel A, Sibbritt D. Risk factors associated with intestinal permeability in an adult population: A systematic review. *Int J Clin Pract.* 2019;73(10):e13385. doi:10.1111/ijcp.13385

238 Janochova K, Haluzik M, Buzga M. Visceral fat and insulin resistance - what we know?. *Biomed Pap Med Fac Univ Palacky Olomouc Czech Repub.* 2019;163(1):19-27. doi:10.5507/bp.2018.062

239 Hyman M. The Doctor's Pharmacy. *The Doctor's Pharmacy.* June 2019. https://drmarkhyman.lnk.to/DrDavidPerlmutter. Accessed April 7, 2020.

240 Sharma, Chetan, et al. "Advanced glycation End-products (AGEs): an emerging concern for processed food industries." *Journal of food science and technology* 52.12 (2015): 7561-7576.

241 Li WW. *Eat to Beat Disease: the New Science of How the Body Can Heal Itself.* New York: Grand Central Publishing; 2019.

242 A. Perfilyev et al., " Impact of Polyunsaturated and Saturated Fat Overfeeding on the DNA-Methylation Pattern in Human Adipose Tissue: A Randomized Controlled Trial," *American Journal of Clinical Nutrition* 105, no. 4 (2017): 991-1000.

243 J. A. Nettleton et al., "Dietary Patterns, Food Groups, and Telomere Length in the Multi-Ethnic Study of Atherosclerosis (MESA)," *American Journal of Clinical Nutrition* 88, no. 5 (2008): 1405-1412.

244 A. M. Fretts et al., "Processed Meat, but Not Unprocessed Red Meat, Is Inversely Associated with Leukocyte Telomere Length in the Strong Heart Family Study," *Journal of Nutrition* 146, no. 10 (2016): 2013-2018.

245 J. A. Nettleton et al., "Dietary Patterns, Food Groups, and Telomere Length in the Multi-Ethnic Study of Atherosclerosis (MESA)," *American Journal of Clinical Nutrition* 88, no. 5 (2008): 1405-1412

246 M. D. Mana, E Y. Kuo, and O. H. Yilmaz, "Dietary Regulation of Adult Stem Cells," *Current Stem Cell Reports* 3, no. 1 (2017): 1-8

247 H. R. Park et al., "A High-Fat Diet Impairs Neurogenesis: Involvement of Lipid Peroxidation and Brain-Derived Neurotrophic Factor," *Neuroscience Letters* 482, no. 3 (2010): 235-239

248 Vafeiadou, Katerina, et al. "A review of the evidence for the effects of total dietary fat, saturated, monounsaturated and n-6 polyunsaturated

fatty acids on vascular function, endothelial progenitor cells and microparticles." *British Journal of Nutrition* 107.3 (2012): 303-324.

[249] Norris, Jill M., et al. "Risk of celiac disease autoimmunity and timing of gluten introduction in the diet of infants at increased risk of disease." *Jama* 293.19 (2005): 2343-2351.

[250] Fasano, Alessio, et al. "Nonceliac gluten sensitivity." *Gastroenterology* 148.6 (2015): 1195-1204.

[251] Eva Bianconi et al., "An Estimation of the Number of Cells in the Human Body," *Annals of Human Biology* 40, no. 6 (2013).

[252] Reyes-Izquierdo, Tania, et al. "Modulatory effect of coffee fruit extract on plasma levels of brain-derived neurotrophic factor in healthy subjects." *British Journal of Nutrition* 110.3 (2013): 420-425.

[253] Zhang ZF, Yang JL, Jiang HC, Lai Z, Wu F, Liu ZX. Updated association of tea consumption and bone mineral density: A meta-analysis. *Medicine (Baltimore)*. 2017;96(12):e6437. doi:10.1097/MD.0000000000006437

[254] H. Sun et al., "The Modulatory Effects of Polyphenols from Green Tea, Oolong Tea, and Black Tea on Human Intestinal Microbiota In Vitro," *Journal of Food Science and Technology* 55, no. 1 (2018): 399-407.

[255] M. Larrosa et al., "Effect of Low Dose of Dietary Resveratrol on Colon Microbiota, Inflammation, and Tissue Damage in a DSS-Induced Colitis Rat Model," *Journal of Agricultural and Food Chemistry* 57, no. 6 (2009): 2211-2220.

[256] A. Jimenez-Giron et al., "Towards the Fecal Metabolome Derived from Moderate Red Wine Intake," *Metabolites* 4, no. 4 (2014): 1101-1118.

[257] D. Wu, J. Wang, M. Pae, and S. N. Meydani, "Green Tea EGCG, T Cells, and T Cell-Mediated Autoimmune Diseases," *Molecular Aspects of Medicine* 33, no. 1 (2012):107-118.

[258] M. R. Olthof, P. C. Hollman, P. L. Zock, and M. B. Katan, "Consumption of High Doses of Chlorogenic Acid, Present in Coffee, or of Black Tea Increases Plasma Total Homocysteine Concentration in Humans," *American Journal of Clinical Nutrition* 73, no. 3 (2001): 532-538.

[259] M. Larrosa et al., "Effect of Low Dose of Dietary Resveratrol on Colon Microbiota, Inflammation, and Tissue Damage in a DSS-Induced Colitis Rat Model," *Journal of Agricultural and Food Chemistry* 57, no. 6 (2009): 2211-2220.

[260] M. M. Markoski et al., "Molecular Properties of Red Wine Compounds and Cardiometabiolic Benefits," *Nutrition and Metabolic Insights* 9 (2016): 51-57

[261] A. Albini et al., "Mechanisms of the Antiangiogenic Activity by the Hop Flavonoid Xanthohumol: NF-kappaB and Akt Targets," *FASEB Journal* 20, no. 3 (2006): 527-529.

[262] M. R. Sartippour et al., "Green Tea Inhibits Vasceular Endothelial Growth Factor (VEGF) Induction in Human Breast Cancer Cells," *Journal of Nutrition* 132, no. 8 (2002): 2307-2311.

[263] Mills CE, Flury A, Marmet C, et al. Mediation of coffee-induced improvements in human vascular function by chlorogenic acids and its metabolites: Two randomized, controlled, crossover intervention trials. *Clin Nutr.* 2017;36(6):1520-1529. doi:10.1016/j.clnu.2016.11.013

[264] W. J. Lee and B. T. Zhu, "Inhibition of DNA Methylation by Caffeic Acid and Chlorogenic Acid, Two Common Catechol-Containing Coffee Polyphenols," *Carcinogenesis* 27, no. 2 (2006): 269-277.

[265] M. Fang, D. Chen, and C. S. Yang, "Dietary Polyphenols May Affect DNA Methylation," *Journal of Nutrition* 137, no. 1 suppl. (2007): 223S-228S.

[266] L. A. Tucker, "Caffeine Consumption and Telomere Length in Men and Women of the National Health and Nutrition Examination Survey (NHANES)," *Nutrition and Metabolism* 14 (2017): 10.

[267] J. J. Liu, M. Crous-Bou, E. Giovannucci, and I. De Vivo, "Coffee Consumption Is Positively Associated with Longer Telomere Length in the Nurses' Health Study," *Journal of Nutrition* 146, no. 7 (2016): 1373-1378

[268] R. Chan et al., "Chinese Tea Consumption is Associated with Longer Telomere Length in Elderly Chinese Men," *British Journal of Nutrition* 146, no. 7 (2010): 107-113

[269] L. Ling, S. Gu, and Y. Cheng, "Resveratrol Activates Endogenous Cardiac Stem Cells and Improve Myocardial Regeneration following Acute Myocardial Infarction," *Molecular Medicine Reports* 15, no. 3 (2017): 1188-1194.

[270] H. L. Kim et al., " Promotion of Full-Thickness Wound Healing Using Epigallocatechiomega-3-O-gallate/Poly(Lactic-co-glycolic Acid) Membrane as Temporary Wound Dressing," *Artficial Organs* 38, no. 5 (2014): 411-417

[271] Y. He et al., "Epigallocatechiomega-3-gallate Attenuates Cerebral Cortex Damage and Promotes Brain Regeneration in Acrylamide-Treated Rate," *Food and Function* 8, no. 6 (2017): 2275-2282

[272] A. R. Kim et al., "Catechins Activate Muscle Stem Cells by Myf5 Induction and Stimulate Muscle Regeneration," *Biochemical and Biophysical Research Communications* 489, no. 2 (2017): 142-148

[273] C. L. Shen et al., "Functions and Mechanisms of Green Tea Catechins in Regulating Bone Remodeling," *Current Drug Targets* 14, no. 13 (2013): 1619-1630

[274] S. Li, H. Bian et al., "Chlorogenic Acid Protects MSCs against Oxidative Stress by Altering FOXO Family Genes and Activating Intrinsic Pathway," *European Journal of Pharmacology* 674, no. 2-3 (2012): 65-72

[275] Komes, Draženka, and Arijana Bušić. "Antioxidants in coffee." *Processing and impact on antioxidants in beverages.* Academic Press, 2014. 25-32.

[276] Rodrigo R, Miranda A, Vergara L. Modulation of endogenous antioxidant system by wine polyphenols in human disease. *Clin Chim Acta.* 2011;412(5-6):410-424. doi:10.1016/j.cca.2010.11.034

[277] Buettner D. *The Blue Zones Solution: Eating and Living like the World's Healthiest People.* Washington, DC: National Geographic Partners; 2017.

[278] "GSTP1 Gene (Protein Coding)," GeneCards Human Gene Database, https://www.genecards.org/cgi-bin/carddisp.pl?gene=GSTP1.

[279] Yokogoshi H, Kobayashi M, Mochizuki M, Terashima T. Effect of theanine, R-glutamylethylamide, on brain monoamines and striatal dopamine release in conscious rats. Neurochem Res 1998;23:667-673.

[280] Yamada T, Terashima T, Kawano S, et al. Theanine, gamma-glutamylethylamide, a unique amino acid in tea leaves, modulates neurotransmitter concentrations in the brain striatum interstitium in conscious rats. Amino Acids 2009;36:21-27

[281] Nobre AC, Rao A, Owen GN. L-theanine, a natural constituent in tea, and its effect on mental state. Asia Pac J Clin Nutr 2008;17:167-168.

[282] Apovian CM. Sugar-sweetened soft drinks, obesity, and type 2 diabetes. JAMA. 2004;292:978-9.

[283] Stärkel P, Leclercq S, de Timary P, Schnabl B. Intestinal dysbiosis and permeability: the yin and yang in alcohol dependence and alcoholic liver disease. Clin Sci (Lond). 2018 Jan 19;132(2):199-212. doi: 10.1042/CS20171055. PMID: 29352076.

[284] Engen PA, Green SJ, Voigt RM, Forsyth CB, Keshavarzian A. The Gastrointestinal Microbiome: Alcohol Effects on the Composition of Intestinal Microbiota. Alcohol Res. 2015;37(2):223-36. PMID: 26695747; PMCID: PMC4590619.

[285] Watson, Ronald R., et al. "Alcohol, immunomodulation, and disease." *Alcohol and alcoholism* 29.2 (1994): 131-139.

[286] Lin WT, Kao YH, Sothern MS, Seal DW, Lee CH, Lin HY, Chen T, Tseng TS. The association between sugar-sweetened beverages intake, body mass index, and inflammation in US adults. Int J Public Health. 2020 Jan;65(1):45-53. doi: 10.1007/s00038-020-01330-5. Epub 2020 Jan 25. PMID: 31982934.

[287] Lu, Yanmin, et al. "Alcohol promotes mammary tumor growth through activation of VEGF-dependent tumor angiogenesis." *Oncology letters* 8.2 (2014): 673-678.

[288] Schiano C, Grimaldi V, Franzese M, Fiorito C, De Nigris F, Donatelli F, Soricelli A, Salvatore M, Napoli C. Non-nutritional sweeteners effects on endothelial vascular function. Toxicol In Vitro. 2020 Feb;62:104694. doi: 10.1016/j.tiv.2019.104694. Epub 2019 Oct 23. PMID: 31655124.

[289] Zakhari S. Alcohol metabolism and epigenetics changes. *Alcohol Res.* 2013;35(1):6-16.

[290] J.A.McClain, D.M. Hayes, S.A. Morris, K. Nixon, "Adolescent Binge Alcohol Exposure Alters Hippocampal Progenitor Cell Proliferation in Rats: Effects on Cell Cycle Kinetics," *Journal of Comparative Neurology* 519, no. 13 (2011): 2697-2710.

[291] Sandhu A, Seth M, Gurm HS
Daylight savings time and myocardial infarction
Open Heart 2014;1:e000019. doi: 10.1136/openhrt-2013-000019

[292] Tononi G, Cirelli C. Sleep and the price of plasticity: from synaptic and cellular homeostasis to memory consolidation and integration. *Neuron.* 2014;81(1):12-34. doi:10.1016/j.neuron.2013.12.025

[293] Raven F, Van der Zee EA, Meerlo P, Havekes R. The role of sleep in regulating structural plasticity and synaptic strength: Implications for memory and cognitive function. *Sleep Med Rev.* 2018;39:3-11. doi:10.1016/j.smrv.2017.05.002

[294] Gingerich SB, Seaverson ELD, Anderson DR. Association Between Sleep and Productivity Loss Among 598 676 Employees From Multiple Industries. *Am J Health Promot.* 2018;32(4):1091-1094. doi:10.1177/0890117117722517

[295] Yin J, Jin X, Shan Z, et al. Relationship of Sleep Duration With All-Cause Mortality and Cardiovascular Events: A Systematic Review and Dose-Response Meta-Analysis of Prospective Cohort Studies. *J Am Heart Assoc.* 2017;6(9):e005947. Published 2017 Sep 9. doi:10.1161/JAHA.117.005947

[296] Burschtin O, Wang J. Testosterone Deficiency and Sleep Apnea. *Sleep Med Clin.* 2016;11(4):525-529. doi:10.1016/j.jsmc.2016.08.003

[297] Abu-Samak MS, Mohammad BA, Abu-Taha MI, Hasoun LZ, Awwad SH. Associations Between Sleep Deprivation and Salivary Testosterone Levels in Male University Students: A Prospective Cohort Study. *Am J Mens Health.* 2018;12(2):411-419. doi:10.1177/1557988317735412

[298] Zhang W, Piotrowska K, Chavoshan B, Wallace J, Liu PY. Sleep Duration Is Associated With Testis Size in Healthy Young Men. *J Clin Sleep Med.* 2018;14(10):1757-1764. Published 2018 Oct 15. doi:10.5664/jcsm.7390

[299] Ding C, Lim LL, Xu L, Kong APS. Sleep and Obesity. *J Obes Metab Syndr.* 2018;27(1):4-24. doi:10.7570/jomes.2018.27.1.4

[300] van Dalfsen JH, Markus CR. The influence of sleep on human hypothalamic-pituitary-adrenal (HPA) axis reactivity: A systematic review. *Sleep Med Rev.* 2018;39:187-194. doi:10.1016/j.smrv.2017.10.002

[301] Holding BC, Sundelin T, Cairns P, Perrett DI, Axelsson J. The effect of sleep deprivation on objective and subjective measures of facial appearance. *J Sleep Res.* 2019;28(6):e12860. doi:10.1111/jsr.12860

[302] Axelsson J, Sundelin T, Ingre M, Van Someren EJ, Olsson A, Lekander M. Beauty sleep: experimental study on the perceived health and attractiveness of sleep deprived people. *BMJ.* 2010;341:c6614. Published 2010 Dec 14. doi:10.1136/bmj.c6614

[303] Simpson NS, Gibbs EL, Matheson GO. Optimizing sleep to maximize performance: implications and recommendations for elite athletes. *Scand J Med Sci Sports.* 2017;27(3):266-274. doi:10.1111/sms.12703

[304] Walker MP. *Why We Sleep: Unlocking the Power of Sleep and Dreams.* New York, NY: Scribner, an imprint of Simon & Schuster, Inc.; 2018.

[305] Irwin MR, Olmstead R, Carroll JE. Sleep Disturbance, Sleep Duration, and Inflammation: A Systematic Review and Meta-Analysis of Cohort Studies and Experimental Sleep Deprivation. *Biol Psychiatry.* 2016;80(1):40-52. doi:10.1016/j.biopsych.2015.05.014

[306] Emil K. Nilsson, Adrian E. Bostrom, Jessica Mwinyi, and Helgi B. Schioth, "Epigenomics of Total Acute Sleep Deprivation in Relation to Genome-Wide DNA Methylation Profiles and RNA Expression," *OMICS* 20, no. 6 (2016): 334-342

[307] G. V. Skuladottir, E. K. Nilsson, J. Mwinyi, and H. B. Schioth, "One-Night Sleep Deprivation Induces Changes in the DNA Methylation and Serum Activity Indices of Stearoyl-CoA Desaturase in Young Healthy Men," *Lipids in Health and Disease* 15, no. 1 (2016): 137.

[308] Jessen NA, Munk AS, Lundgaard I, Nedergaard M. The Glymphatic System: A Beginner's Guide. *Neurochem Res.* 2015;40(12):2583-2599. doi:10.1007/s11064-015-1581-6

[309] Cai, Denise J., et al. "REM, not incubation, improves creativity by priming associative networks." *Proceedings of the National Academy of Sciences* 106.25 (2009): 10130-10134.

[310] van Dalfsen JH, Markus CR. The influence of sleep on human hypothalamic-pituitary-adrenal (HPA) axis reactivity: A systematic review. *Sleep Med Rev.* 2018;39:187-194. doi:10.1016/j.smrv.2017.10.002

[311] Walker MP. *Why We Sleep: Unlocking the Power of Sleep and Dreams.* New York, NY: Scribner, an imprint of Simon & Schuster, Inc.; 2018.

[312] Goodwin, Renee D., and Andrej Marusic. "Association between short sleep and suicidal ideation and suicide attempt among adults in the general population." *Sleep* 31.8 (2008): 1097-1101.

[313] CLEAR JAMES. *ATOMIC HABITS: an Easy and Proven Way to Build Good Habits and Break Bad Ones.* Place of publication not identified: RANDOM House BUSINESS; 2019.

[314] Buettner D. *The Blue Zones: 9 Lessons for Living Longer from the People Whove Lived the Longest.* Washington, D.C.: National Geographic; 2012.

[315] Hargrove T. *Playing With Movement.* Better Movement; 2019.

[316] Erickson, Kirk I., et al. "Exercise training increases size of hippocampus and improves memory." *Proceedings of the National Academy of Sciences* 108.7 (2011): 3017-3022.

[317] Yogman M, Garner A, Hutchinson J, et al. The Power of Play: A Pediatric Role in Enhancing Development in Young Children. *Pediatrics.* 2018;142(3):e20182058. doi:10.1542/peds.2018-2058

[318] Mailing, Lucy J., et al. "Exercise and the gut microbiome: a review of the evidence, potential mechanisms, and implications for human health." *Exercise and sport sciences reviews* 47.2 (2019): 75-85.

[319] Chinsomboon, Jessica, et al. "The transcriptional coactivator PGC-1α mediates exercise-induced angiogenesis in skeletal muscle." *Proceedings of the national academy of sciences* 106.50 (2009): 21401-21406.

[320] M. Du et al., "Physical Activity, Sedentary Behavior, and Leukocyte Telomere Length in Women," *American Journal of Epidemiology* 175, no. 5 (2012): 414-422

[321] D. Ornish et al., "Increased Telomerase Activity and Comprehensive Lifestyle Changes: A Pilot Study," *Lancet Oncology* 9, no. 11 (2008): 1048-1057.

[322] He, Congcong, Rhea Sumpter, Jr, and Beth Levine. "Exercise induces autophagy in peripheral tissues and in the brain." *Autophagy* 8.10 (2012): 1548-1551.

[323] Brandt N, Gunnarsson TP, Bangsbo J, Pilegaard H. Exercise and exercise training-induced increase in autophagy markers in human skeletal muscle. *Physiol Rep.* 2018;6(7):e13651. doi:10.14814/phy2.13651

[324] Etnier JL, Wideman L, Labban JD, et al. The Effects of Acute Exercise on Memory and Brain-Derived Neurotrophic Factor (BDNF). *J Sport Exerc Psychol.* 2016;38(4):331-340. doi:10.1123/jsep.2015-0335

[325] Maass A, Düzel S, Brigadski T, et al. Relationships of peripheral IGF-1, VEGF and BDNF levels to exercise-related changes in memory, hippocampal perfusion and volumes in older adults. *Neuroimage.* 2016;131:142-154. doi:10.1016/j.neuroimage.2015.10.084

[326] de Sousa CV, Sales MM, Rosa TS, Lewis JE, de Andrade RV, Simões HG. The Antioxidant Effect of Exercise: A Systematic Review and Meta-Analysis. *Sports Med.* 2017;47(2):277-293. doi:10.1007/s40279-016-0566-1

[327] Lim SA, Cheong KJ. Regular Yoga Practice Improves Antioxidant Status, Immune Function, and Stress Hormone Releases in Young Healthy People: A Randomized, Double-Blind, Controlled Pilot Study. *J Altern Complement Med.* 2015;21(9):530-538. doi:10.1089/acm.2014.0044

[328] Stonerock GL, Hoffman BM, Smith PJ, Blumenthal JA. Exercise as Treatment for Anxiety: Systematic Review and Analysis. *Ann Behav Med.* 2015;49(4):542-556. doi:10.1007/s12160-014-9685-9

[329] Rubio-Arias JÁ, Marín-Cascales E, Ramos-Campo DJ, Hernandez AV, Pérez-López FR. Effect of exercise on sleep quality and insomnia in middle-aged women: A systematic review and meta-analysis of randomized controlled trials. *Maturitas.* 2017;100:49-56. doi:10.1016/j.maturitas.2017.04.003

[330] Buettner D. Thrive: Finding Happiness the Blue Zones Way: Seven Secrets from the World's Happiest People. Washington, D.C.: National Geographic; 2010.

[331] Buettner D. The Blue Zones: 9 Lessons for Living Longer from the People Who've Lived the Longest. Washington, D.C.: National Geographic; 2012.

[332] Leigh-Hunt N, Bagguley D, Bash K, et al. An overview of systematic reviews on the public health consequences of social isolation and loneliness. *Public Health.* 2017;152:157-171. doi:10.1016/j.puhe.2017.07.035

[333] Steptoe A, Shankar A, Demakakos P, Wardle J. Social isolation, loneliness, and all-cause mortality in older men and women. *Proceedings of the National Academy of Sciences.* 2013;110(15):5797-5801. doi:10.1073/pnas.1219686110.

[334] Shankar, A., McMunn, A., Banks, J., & Steptoe, A. (2011). Loneliness, social isolation, and behavioral and biological health indicators in older adults. *Health Psychology*, 30(4), 377–385. https://doi.org/10.1037/a0022826

[335] Friends and Family May Play a Role in Obesity. National Institutes of Health. https://www.nih.gov/news-events/nih-research-matters/friends-family-may-play-role-obesity. Published July 6, 2015. Accessed April 15, 2020.

[336] Moeller AH, Foerster S, Wilson ML, Pusey AE, Hahn BH, Ochman H. Social behavior shapes the chimpanzee pan-microbiome. Sci Adv. 2016 Jan 15;2(1):e1500997. doi: 10.1126/sciadv.1500997. PMID: 26824072; PMCID: PMC4730854.

[337] Shankar, A., McMunn, A., Banks, J., & Steptoe, A. (2011). Loneliness, social isolation, and behavioral and biological health indicators in older adults. *Health Psychology*, 30(4), 377–385. https://doi.org/10.1037/a0022826

[338] Cacioppo, J.T., & Hawkley, L.C. (2003). Social Isolation and Health, with an Emphasis on Underlying Mechanisms. *Perspectives in Biology and Medicine* 46(3), S39-S52. doi:10.1353/pbm.2003.0049.

[339] Inspired by: Buettner D. Thrive: Finding Happiness the Blue Zones Way: Seven Secrets from the World's Happiest People. Washington, D.C.: National Geographic; 2010.

[340] Wei Q, Lee JH, Wang H, et al. Adiponectin is required for maintaining normal body temperature in a cold environment. BMC Physiol. 2017;17(1):8. Published 2017 Oct 23. doi:10.1186/s12899-017-0034-7

[341] Fenzl A, Kiefer FW. Brown adipose tissue and thermogenesis. Horm Mol Biol Clin Investig. 2014;19(1):25-37. doi:10.1515/hmbci-2014-0022

[342] Heinonen I, Laukkanen JA. Effects of heat and cold on health, with special reference to Finnish sauna bathing. Am J Physiol Regul Integr Comp Physiol. 2018;314(5):R629-R638. doi:10.1152/ajpregu.00115.2017

[343] Kukkonen-Harjula, K., and K. Kauppinen. "How the sauna affects the endocrine system." *Annals of Clinical Research* 20.4 (1988): 262.

[344] Raison CL, Knight JM, Pariante C. Interleukin (IL)-6: A good kid hanging out with bad friends (and why sauna is good for health). *Brain Behav Immun.* 2018;73:1-2. doi:10.1016/j.bbi.2018.06.008

[345] Heinonen I, Laukkanen JA. Effects of heat and cold on health, with special reference to Finnish sauna bathing. Am J Physiol Regul Integr Comp Physiol. 2018;314(5):R629-R638. doi:10.1152/ajpregu.00115.2017

[346] N. S. Schutte and J. M. Malouff, " A Meta-Analytic Review of the Effects of Mindfulness Meditation on Telomerase Activity," *Psychoneuroendocrinology* 42 (2014): 45-48.

[347] P. Kaliman et al., "Rapid Changes in Histone Deacetylases and Inflammatory Gene Espression in Expert Meditators," *Psychoneuroendocrinology* 40 (2014): 96-107

[348] Rao KS, Chakraharti SK, Dongare VS, et al. Antiaging Effects of an Intensive Mind and Body Therapeutic Program through Enhancement of Telomerase Activity and Adult Stem Cell Counts. J Stem Cells. 2015;10(2):107-125.

[349] Rubin BS. Bisphenol A: an endocrine disruptor with widespread exposure and multiple effects. J Steroid Biochem Mol Biol. 2011 Oct;127(1-2):27-34. doi: 10.1016/j.jsbmb.2011.05.002. Epub 2011 May 13. PMID: 21605673.

[350] Sanchez de Badajoz E, Lage-Sánchez JM, Sánchez-Gallegos P. Endocrine disruptors and prostate cancer. Arch Esp Urol. 2017 Apr;70(3):331-335. English, Spanish. PMID: 28422034.

[351] Kabir ER, Rahman MS, Rahman I. A review on endocrine disruptors and their possible impacts on human health. Environ Toxicol Pharmacol. 2015 Jul;40(1):241-58. doi: 10.1016/j.etap.2015.06.009. Epub 2015 Jun 9. PMID: 26164742.

352 Cook G. *Movement: Functional Movement Systems: Screening, Assessment and Corrective Strategies*. Santa Cruz, CA: On Target Publications; 2017.

353 Cook G. *Athletic Body in Balance*. Champaign, IL: Human Kinetics; 2005.

354 Liebenson C. *Functional Training Handbook*. Philadelphia: Wolters Kluwer Health; 2014.

355 Corre EL. *The Practice of Natural Movement: Reclaim Power, Health, and Freedom*. Auberry, Calif. USA: Victory Belt Publishing Inc.; 2019.

356 Starrett K, Cordoza G. *Becoming a Supple Leopard: the Ultimate Guide to Resolving Pain, Preventing Injury, and Optimizing Athletic Performance*. Las Vegas, NV: Victory Belt Publishing; 2015.

357 Brito LB, Ricardo DR, Araújo DS, Ramos PS, Myers J, Araújo CG. Ability to sit and rise from the floor as a predictor of all-cause mortality. Eur J Prev Cardiol. 2014 Jul;21(7):892-8. doi: 10.1177/2047487312471759. Epub 2012 Dec 13. PMID: 23242910.

Made in the USA
Columbia, SC
24 April 2021